MINDFIRE

MINDFIRE

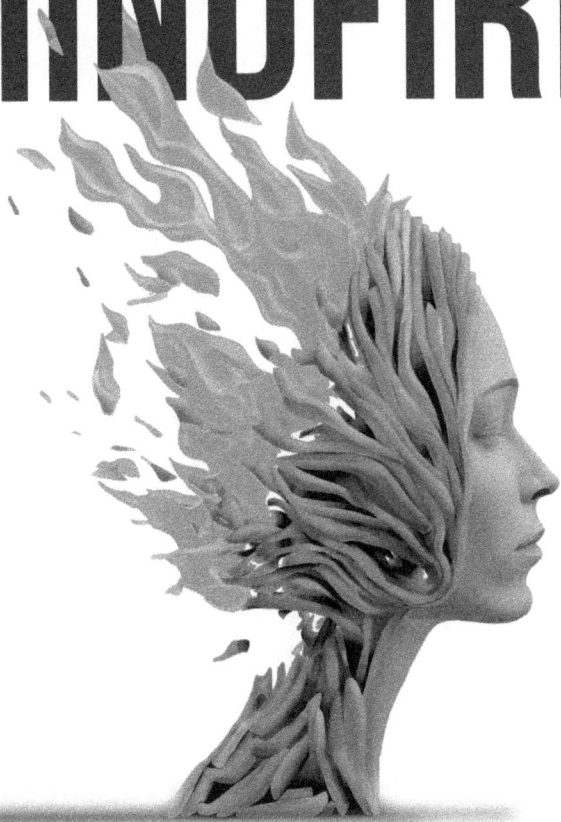

The Surprising Science of How
Brain Inflammation Impacts Mental Health,
and What You Can Do About It

XENIA KACHUR
AND LUKE STARBUCK

LIONCREST
PUBLISHING

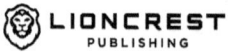

MINDFIRE
*The Surprising Science of How Brain Inflammation Impacts
Mental Health, and What You Can Do About It*

FIRST EDITION

ISBN   978-1-5445-4578-3   *Hardcover*
       978-1-5445-4576-9   *Paperback*
       978-1-5445-4577-6   *Ebook*

This book is dedicated to every person who
believes a better quality of life is possible.

CONTENTS

DISCLAIMER

This book provides general information based on recent research and is for informational purposes only. Neither the author nor the publisher are healthcare professionals. This book is not a source of medical advice. Always consult with a healthcare provider for medical concerns. The suggestions herein are based on research and personal insights and should not replace professional medical guidance.

The author and publisher expressly disclaim responsibility for any adverse events or outcomes that may result from the use or application of the information contained in this book.

INTRODUCTION

It was a perfect, blue-sky day. From where we were, halfway up our climb, we could see the whole valley laid out below us, the river winding between the steep, red rock cliffs. We were at Smith Rock State Park in Oregon, rock climbing a route up the steep face of a mountain. My friend and I took turns who would climb each section first, and then the other would follow.

A little over halfway up the mountain face, my friend climbed away from me on one of the harder sections. He was out of sight for a long time, the only signal from him an occasional tug on the rope. Eventually, he made it to the next stopping point, and I started to climb.

I was connected to a rope, tied to my partner above me and attached to the rock. So maybe I wasn't as careful as I could have been. Or maybe I was weighed down by the pack full of gear I was carrying with me. Whatever happened, I reached for a hold, lost my grip, and fell.

I had only gotten about 15 feet above the ledge I'd started climbing from, and the rope we were using was stretchy enough that it didn't break any of the 15-foot fall. I landed, hard, on my back on a giant rock sitting on the cliff's edge. It was a lucky thing I was carrying the pack, since it protected my back from the worst of the fall. But it also bent me backward, whipping my head.

Right away, I could tell the injury was bad. I was pretty sure I had a concussion and probably a broken tailbone as well. I was in pain and disoriented.

My friend was too far above me to hear me scream. He had no idea what had happened. It would be farther to try to climb back down than to go up. I had no choice. I started climbing again.

I made it up the 200 feet to where my friend was, and together, we made it the rest of the way to the top of the route and off the mountain. Unfortunately, that wasn't the end of my problems. In fact, it was only the beginning.

Within a few days of the accident, I wasn't sleeping through the night. I would fall asleep, but then wake up, *fully* awake, every few hours and struggle to get back to sleep. After just a few days of that, coupled with brain fog and disorientation, I was completely wrecked. Then I started feeling extreme anxiety and panic at random times during the day. I needed to do something about it.

When I went to the doctor, he confirmed that I had a concussion. When I asked him what I could do about it, all he said was, "Sit in a dark room, and avoid stress."

I stopped working. I stopped socializing. I pretty much just stayed at home and read sci-fi books and hoped I was getting better. But over the next few months, I didn't get better. If anything, I kept getting worse. I could barely leave the house. I couldn't be around people for very long. Despite having been a very active person before, now I couldn't walk my dogs around the block without sitting down to rest multiple times. No matter how long I sat in the dark, nothing was changing.

I assumed something was seriously wrong with me, like a brain tumor or an immune disease, so I went to see a neurologist. He took an MRI brain scan and informed me, "There's nothing serious here, nothing that I can see."

"But I'm not getting better," I said. "My symptoms are debilitating. I can't think properly. I can't even drive!"

He wrote his prescription for what I should do—*no stress, no screens*—and sent me out the door.

A second neurologist offered me medications for the symptoms: medications for my anxiety, medications for sleep. He told me to reduce my stress. For months, all I did was stay home. I didn't have the focus to drive safely. I was living in a haze of brain fog. My symptoms already filled two typed pages, and I wasn't willing to add pharmaceutical side effects to it. I didn't want a Band-Aid for my symptoms. I needed to heal my brain.

I decided enough was enough and started looking for my own answers.

Luckily for me, I had a background in biomedical engineering. I found every single scientific research paper I could find that dealt with symptoms like mine. I read hundreds of papers, looking for anything that could help.

And then I started trying things. I tried biofeedback. Chinese medicine. Hyperbaric oxygen. Cold plunging. Things I'd never heard of and common approaches I hadn't previously realized were so strongly supported by evidence. I tried everything that had strong science to back it up.

And after a few months, there came a day when I woke up and I felt...*good*. At that point, I barely remembered what "good" felt like. I felt like I could breathe again.

I went back to my medical team, excited to tell them about what I'd done. I told them about the approaches I'd tried and how much better I felt.

I got a lot of blank looks and distracted nods. They'd heard of some of the things I was talking about, but they'd never used any of them. And some of them they had never even heard of, despite decades of supporting research.

That made me ask myself: *What else is there?* What else might help me? What else did my team of specialists not yet know about?

It turns out, there was a lot more. A lot more out there that could help me—and maybe you too. Even if you've never had a concussion or noticeable illness that affected your brain.

WHO AM I TO SAY?

If even my neurologists hadn't heard of these approaches, why should you listen to me? How can you know that these are things you should try?

One reason is that I've been where you are, tried most of these things for myself, and found that they work.

The other reason is that these aren't methods I came up with. I'm not a doctor or a medical scientist. I am trained to understand and evaluate scientific evidence though.

And I'm very, very motivated.

Doctors are motivated to help their patients get better. But they are also very busy. They can't possibly keep up with every single research study that comes out about every single symptom or condition. They tend to focus on whatever is in their own field of study, whether that's neurology or surgery. Anything outside that, they don't seek out.

I didn't have that limitation. I wanted—*needed*—to get better, so I looked at everything. Neuroscience and medical studies, sure, but also studies about meditation, breathing exercises, nutrition, sleep... you name it. If it showed promise in people with symptoms like mine, I read it, evaluated it, and if the science was strong, I tried it.

That means that I'm standing on the shoulders of literally thousands of researchers in dozens of fields of study, not to mention hundreds of years of practitioners using everything from yoga to saunas. If you want to know more about where the information in this book comes from, feel free to flip to the back and check out the hundreds of studies I've referenced. Don't worry, though. The point of this book is that you don't need to go find all those studies and figure it out for yourself.

Each chapter gives you the most important information you need to know about the research, then helps you make sense of that and apply it to improve your own mental health and quality of life.

If you're where I was, that should make figuring out what to do to feel better a whole lot easier.

ARE YOU STRUGGLING TOO?

The more I learned about what was going on with me, the more I understood that it went far beyond the one concussion.

The long-term, debilitating symptoms I was suffering from were the result of many experiences over the course of my entire life. PTSD. Long-term anxiety. Childhood trauma. The head injuries magnified all these things, but my poor mental health was a result of all of them combined.

The more research I did, and the more methods I tried, the more I found out that I was not alone.

Many of us are suffering from these issues, and often, we don't even know it.

If you've been living with a mental health issue for a long time, it can become part of your everyday experience. It almost becomes background. You're tired all the time, or you can't focus when you need to. Your head never seems totally clear. You've got aches and pains all over your body without any clear reason why. Maybe you jump at the slightest noises or get anxious as soon as you have to interact with other people.

Maybe you've gone back to doctor after doctor, trying to get answers and being told it's "just stress" or even that there's "nothing wrong." Maybe you've struggled with anxiety or what feels like depression, but you don't want to use medications.

If so, this book is for you.

It's also for you if you have tried some of the more common methods of treating mental health issues and been unsatisfied. If you're a person who's not content with "Band-Aid" solutions, and wants instead to get to the heart of a problem and understand it, you will find answers here.

I can't diagnose what is going on with you. That's something you need a medical or mental health provider for.

What I can do is share with you the evidence-based, scientifically validated methods that can help you start to gain control back in your own life.

INFLAMED

This book is about something called inflammation. Inflammation is a normal part of the body's response to stress, injury, or illness.

We'll spend lots of time later in the book on what inflammation is and how it works. The key is that new science shows that when inflammation gets out of control—especially *brain* inflammation—it's connected with tons of different kinds of mental and cognitive health problems.

Problems like anxiety. Depression. PTSD.

Symptoms like brain fog. Sleeplessness. Fatigue.

Everywhere I turned in my research, inflammation kept coming up. It's been tied to Alzheimer's disease and multiple sclerosis and Parkinson's. It's connected to sleep disorders and migraines and learning difficulties.

The thing is, *your brain is your life.* What I mean by that is, your brain is the lens you see everything else through. It's how you feel. How you interpret the things that happen to you. How you make sense of the world. So when that lens is foggy or warped or smudged for whatever reason, it affects your entire life.

When I made that connection, that my mental health was dependent on my *brain* health, that's when things started to change for me. It's when I started investigating the role of inflammation and finding out how key it was to my brain's experience of the world.

If you are struggling with mental health issues, there's a very good chance inflammation is involved.

The upside is that there are many scientifically backed ways to reduce that inflammation and get your quality of life back.

HOW THIS BOOK WORKS

The book is organized so that you're introduced to the background information first—the science of inflammation—and then the different approaches.

But you don't have to read it that way. Feel free to skip around. You might want to know the basics first and understand the biology of your body and what's happening to you. Or you might want to skip straight to everyday changes you can make or even right to the bioaccelerators at the end of the book.

Read it in any order that makes sense to you. And if the science gets too dense or complex, feel free to skip it. The important takeaway remains the same: what to *do* to improve your mental health and your life.

Section One of this book will introduce you to inflammation: what it is and how it shows up in your body. I'll show you what inflammation looks like when it's doing its job—and what happens when it flares out of control. You'll also meet a number of people who are living with inflammation-related conditions, whose stories we'll follow throughout the book.

Section Two introduces everyday lifestyle adjustments you can make to start fighting inflammation. The food you eat, how and how much you move your body, and how you sleep can all affect your mental and brain health through inflammation. In each case, these everyday behaviors can be positive (fighting inflammation) or negative (causing inflammation or making it worse). I'll give you the information to make positive choices.

Section Three takes you through the most commonly used approaches to mental health: medications (including supplements), therapy, and "alternative" practices like yoga and mindfulness. Most people who have experienced mental health problems will have tried, or at least been encouraged to try, one or all of these options. And while medications, therapy, and alternative medicine can all be important tools in your anti-inflammatory toolbox, you need to be cautious about what you're taking or trying, and why.

Finally, **Section Four** introduces what I call the bioaccelerators: methods and approaches that exponentially speed up or activate the natural healing mechanisms in your body. We'll talk about psychedelics, which are proving to be some of the most potent anti-inflammatory medicines we have. Then I'll introduce you to a number of exciting new technologies that are being used to treat even the most long-term, previously untreatable mental health issues.

Every chapter ends with a tl;dr section (that stands for "too long; didn't read"). These summary sections highlight the key points to take away with you.

INFORMED CHOICE, NOT "SELF-HELP"

The purpose of this book isn't exactly "self-help." Yes, I'm going to introduce you to lifestyle tools you can use to reduce inflammation and improve your quality of life. But a lot of the approaches and methods outlined here require a professional (like a doctor or a mental health practitioner) or access to technologies that you probably don't have at home.

The important difference between "self-help" and "informed choices" is that a self-help book says, *Try this—it will work!* (Usually because it worked for the person who wrote the book.) And that's great.

Informed choice is different. It's me telling you, *Here are the latest, most exciting scientific findings and new methods for treating symptoms you might not even have realized were treatable!* And then you decide which tools, approaches, or combinations are right for your individual situation.

There are literally *dozens* of approaches in this book to choose from. Some you can do in your living room. Others require a medical doctor or a piece of high-tech equipment.

You can pick and choose, change your mind later, or try a bunch of different things. I'm not telling you, "Do this." I'm showing you: "Look what is possible."

For those of us living with mental health problems that are weighing us down, reducing our quality of life, and making us wonder whether we can ever get better, just the news that *real, evidence-based methods exist* can be life-changing in itself.

The point is this: *better is out there.* However you're feeling, there are ways to feel better. The science is out there. The technologies are out there. It's just a matter of getting access to the information and the right tools.

That starts with understanding inflammation and how it can help—and harm—your body and your mind.

FROM ADVERSITY TO INSIGHT

CHAPTER ONE

———

THE MANY FACES OF INFLAMMATION

Inflamed: hot, fiery, flaming, aroused, raging, smoldering, burning

It was 2015, and I was sitting in yet another doctor's office. My head was pounding under the fluorescent lights as I listened to the same old stuff I'd been told over and over again: Get more rest. Try to limit your screen time. Work on reducing your stress.

No kidding, I thought. *I would love to reduce my stress. Except that it's hard to be less stressed when your anxiety is pushing your heartbeat through your ears and your depression is making it hard to get out of bed. I would love to get more rest too. Too bad I haven't been able to sleep through the night for six months.*

When I told my doctors about these problems, there were a lot of them they couldn't do anything about at all. For the others, all they could offer me was pills. Drugs to help me sleep. Drugs to reduce anxiety. Drugs for depression. Drugs for my memory problems so I wouldn't forget to take the others.

Of course, every single one of those drugs came with its own list of side effects. Some of the side effects were symptoms I already had, or worse. Given the two-page list of symptoms I was already experiencing, this wasn't a gamble I was willing to take.

I was suffering, just like you might be suffering if you picked up this book. Every day was a fight with fatigue and brain fog and depression. Every night was another desperate attempt to get enough sleep to make it through another day.

But I was also lucky. I was trained as a biomedical engineer, so I knew how to read and understand scientific research. If my doctors couldn't offer me any other options, maybe I could find a solution myself. I started learning everything I could about the symptoms I was having—and why they wouldn't go away.

I dove into the newest research, desperate for something that might fix what was happening to me.

I tried everything from traditional remedies to experimental, high-tech approaches. Acupuncture, hydrotherapy, supplements and interval training, sensory deprivation tanks, dialectical behavioral therapy, hyperbaric oxygen pods—anything I could get my hands on. I became my own guinea pig. If an option had science behind it, I was willing to give it a chance. For three years, I kept at it.

Every time I tried a new approach, I asked myself, *Is this helping? Am I getting better?*

The answer, miraculously, was *yes*.

With these new approaches, I was finally improving. I hadn't even realized how bad the fog was until it started to lift. For the first time in years, I was not having difficulty remembering things at work. Depression wasn't pulling me under every time I made a step forward. *I was getting myself back.*

I also realized that many, many other people must be suffering from the same types of life-altering symptoms I was experiencing. Mine started with a concussion, but others were experiencing the same problems as a result of long-term stress, traumatic experiences, major illness, or other kinds of injuries. Some of them went to their doctors for depression or anxiety, while others were diagnosed with autoimmune diseases or memory problems or sleeplessness. Often, they were told that these problems were just part of "getting older" or "postmenopausal changes."

The more I researched all these conditions and their causes, the more I kept seeing one word show up again and again.

Inflammation.

THE FIRE INSIDE

Inflammation has gotten a lot of press lately. You might have heard about it from your doctor or seen posts about it on Instagram. If you know someone with arthritis, or if you've ever been really ill with an infection, you might have been told something about inflammation. You might know that it's a natural process in your body that occurs when you're injured or stressed or ill.

But that's only a small part of the picture.

What has just been understood very recently is that inflammation can get out of control, and when that happens, the effects can take over your life. Pain, depression, brain fog, insomnia, memory problems, headaches, fatigue, autoimmune diseases—the list of conditions that can be caused or worsened by inflammation goes on and on.

If you look at the word itself, you can see why. "Inflammation" has the same origin as the word "flame." So when inflammation gets out of hand, it's like a fire burning in your body, brain, and mind.

Fire is a strange thing. It kills and destroys, but it's also necessary for life.

Take a forest fire, for example. Weeds and brush that grow too big are like ropes binding and choking the forest. When lightning ignites a spark, the fire burns the excess away, letting the forest breathe again. Charred plants become food for living ones. Mushrooms thrust up from the cleared ground. The rain seeps deeper into the soil. Fire is necessary for the forest ecosystem to thrive. It's part of a healthy cycle, even if it's harmful in the short term.

But what if the fire never stopped?

What if the fire kept burning? What if it burned through the hardest hardwood trees and ate healthy branches as well as dead ones? What if flames scorched the green leaves and left the trees gasping for breath and unable to recover? What if the fire simply raged on for years? The natural processes of recovery would be strained past their limits. The forest would exhaust itself in the struggle to survive.

Whenever you're injured or ill, your immune system acts like a forest fire, killing and burning away the intruders. That's inflammation. It's a healthy and important part of how your body responds to harm.

When the inflammation has done its work, your body heals. Like the forest, your body recovers. But sometimes, for lots of reasons I'll get into later, the immune response never gets shut off. The fire keeps burning. It turns its heat on healthy cells and tissues and causes damage.

When the immune response doesn't get turned off, it's called chronic inflammation. "Chronic" refers to a situation that continues for a long time or keeps coming back. Chronic inflammation can cause or magnify a huge range of symptoms and long-term illnesses that scientists and doctors didn't even realize were related until very recently.

So what happens when the fire in your body and brain doesn't go out? In this chapter, I'm going to show you some of the ways chronic inflammation can look and feel. You might be surprised by how many different ways it can show up, from depression and anxiety to brain fog and chronic pain. Like me, you might see your own issues and symptoms in these stories.

If that happens, don't worry. Knowing what's gone wrong is the first step toward healing.

THE MANY FACES OF INFLAMMATION

One of the reasons it's so hard to understand and treat chronic inflammation is that it has many unique faces.

It's pretty easy for your doctor to diagnose a common condition like a strep throat or an obvious physical injury like a broken bone. If you've got a sore throat, for example, the doctor can swab your throat and run a simple test that will tell her whether you have strep. Your symptoms might not be exactly identical to everyone else's, but it's clear what is going on in your body.

When you're feeling brain fog, or you're more anxious than you're used to, things get more challenging.

Inflammation—especially chronic inflammation that hasn't been treated—doesn't work that way. It can look very different in different people. That's why it's taken decades for scientists to realize that so many seemingly different conditions have this same underlying factor.

Plus, we're just discovering that chronic inflammation can have a lot more causes than anyone imagined. Inflammation can be the result of something that just happened recently, like an illness or an injury. It can be a response to something that's a regular part of our everyday lives, like work stress. Stranger still, it can also be the result of something that happened *decades* ago, like childhood trauma.

If inflammation is a wildfire, these events are like lightning strikes that set it ablaze. And just like with wildfires, it can be hard to figure out the cause once the fire is already burning.

We'll talk a lot more about the science of inflammation in later chapters, along with what you can do if you discover that chronic inflammation is causing your symptoms. First, though, I'd like to briefly introduce you to a few people who are living with chronic inflammation in its many forms.

Their stories, their lives, and their symptoms are all different—at least on the surface. But incredible as it seems, all of their conditions are caused by that one common enemy: chronic inflammation.

You'll be learning more about them later in the book. You'll hear about their situations, their treatment journeys, and the methods they used to get back to a higher quality of life. For now, just take in the incredibly varied ways that out-of-control inflammation can look, and feel, in different people's lives.

Each of these stories captures the struggles and successes of real people I've worked with in my brain fitness center. For privacy and to keep the stories relevant, I've combined different people's experiences into these stories. None of these are real, individual people. But they tell real people's stories, nonetheless.

Camilla is a psychotherapist in her early 40s. Camilla suffered a difficult upbringing as the child of refugees. She was diagnosed with fibromyalgia seven years ago, and now she is really struggling. Every day, she wakes up with pain and fatigue. She often gets little or no sleep. She's trying hard to keep her psychotherapy practice going, but the stiffness and pain in her body seem to just keep getting worse. It's also getting harder to hide the fact that she has trouble remembering things that happened yesterday or last week.

Jadyn is a student in his late 20s. He's a barista during the day and attends online coding school at night. Recently, he's having a lot of trouble concentrating and feeling motivated. It's like he just can't learn as fast as he used to. At the café where he works, he keeps making rookie mistakes, putting the wrong ingredients in drinks he knows how to make and forgetting orders in the middle of making them. Jadyn just can't figure out what's wrong. He's always had tons of energy. He's the life of the party! But now, he can barely drag himself through his day. Sure, he had COVID-19 a few months ago, but aside from a week off work, he barely noticed it. Whatever's wrong with him now seems to be different—and it's getting worse rather than better.

Stephanie is a mom of three teenagers. She loves her life. The problem is that everything has become overwhelming. She used to be able to coach her son's ultimate frisbee team, pick up her daughter from swimming, make dinner, and help with homework. No sweat. Then five years ago, she was in a car accident. That's when everything changed. At first it was stuff she could understand. Panic attacks while she was driving. Feeling like lights are too bright and sounds are too loud. She thought it was anxiety from the accident, so she tried therapy and then yoga. Nothing seemed to be working. Now, *her list of concerns is growing. She's started having stomach issues too. Life is starting to feel unmanageable.*

Ash has always been a go-getter. In accounting school, they were always at the top of their class. Now, at only 37, they have just been offered a fast track to a major promotion at the accounting firm where they work. It's a big raise and a lot more responsibility. Even though that's what Ash has been working toward, it's a little scary. Ash has suffered from depression on and off since their teen years, when they first started experiencing gender identity discrimination. They have also had migraines since they were 16. Usually, the migraines only come about once a month, but recently, it's been more like once or twice a week. Ash long ago learned how to work through the vomiting-level pain, but the tricks they once used don't seem to be working anymore. Part of it is life on the road. Ash spends almost as much time traveling to visit clients as they do at home. The client meetings and the high-profile work are great, but the thousands of restaurant meals and hotel rooms seem to be catching up. Ash is becoming very afraid that even if they're offered that promotion, they may have to turn it down after all.

Childhood trauma. COVID-19. PTSD. Work stress. Aren't these all separate, unrelated problems?

Yes. And incredibly enough, also no.

Every one of these conditions and events can cause inflammation. If the inflammation is left untreated, it can cause symptoms years or even decades later.

Treating all of these conditions as if they're totally separate ignores the critical, powerful role of inflammation in our mental and physical well-being.

THE INFLAMMATION EMERGENCY

Are you ready to be shocked? Here's a *partial* list of the conditions and symptoms that can have inflammation as a major factor:

Anxiety	Depression	Sleep Problems
Memory Problems	Hypervigilance	Concentration Problems
Brain Fog	Irritability	Mood Imbalances
Fatigue	Dizziness	Arthritis
Cancer	Diabetes	Alzheimer's
Heart Disease	Chronic Pain	Stroke
Hyper/hypothyroidism	Parkinson's	Multiple Sclerosis

That's a lot of different conditions—and those are just the physical problems. Think about the effects on individual lives. Missed work, missed opportunities, lowered quality of life, loss of enjoyment, strained relationships, isolation...the list goes on and on.

Even the smallest-seeming symptoms can cause major changes that can steal our quality of life, especially if they go on and on for years. If you're too dizzy to climb up into the stands, do you miss your daughter's softball game? If you're irritable all the time, how long will your spouse put up with it? Just like inflammation can build up over time, the effects of "minor" symptoms can grow until they diminish or even degrade your quality of life.

Given all of this, I don't think I'm exaggerating when I say that chronic inflammation is an emergency. When it's happening to you, it certainly feels like one.

So how come you don't already know about it? Why isn't this common knowledge?

There are a lot of reasons. One of them is your skull.

PROGRESS IN BRAIN SCIENCE...FINALLY

Your skull is there to protect you. To make sure your fragile, all-important brain, the home of all your thoughts and feelings, isn't easily injured.

Your head is the exact opposite of the rest of your body. Most of your body has soft tissues like skin and muscle on the outside, with the hard, dense skeleton underneath. Because your brain is so important, the dense skull is on the outside instead, like armor. Which is great for protection but not so great for looking inside.

As if that doesn't make it hard enough, your skull is also full of liquid. Right inside your skull is a membrane, like a balloon. That balloon is full of fluid (called *cerebrospinal fluid*). Your brain floats around in that liquid.

I know, it sounds kind of gross. But stay with me.

The point of this layered system is protection. Your brain is soft and easily damaged. If it were loose inside your skull, the slightest motion could smash it up against the hard bone and damage it. The balloon full of liquid is a soft container, allowing your brain to move around without hitting the skull.

Well, usually. A concussion is what happens when the brain moves so much that it gets jolted into the skull and damaged. So you can see why it's important to keep the brain floating and safe.

Here's the problem: your brain is so well protected that it's really difficult to study.

Almost everyone has heard of MRIs and CT scans: imaging technologies that can give you a detailed picture of what's going wrong in your body. But what if what's wrong is smaller than what the technologies can see? If you tear your ACL, an MRI is great. It can see the structural details of where you tore it and provide necessary insights to the surgeon on how to fix it.

Using these tools to image the brain can tell you if there's serious damage to its physical structure (like a tumor, or internal bleeding from an accident). But they can't tell you what's causing your thoughts and feelings. This is because there are a lot of processes happening on a very small scale: at the cellular and molecular levels. Trying to see a molecular process using a CT scan is like trying to locate a penny on your roof using Google Earth satellite footage. It's just not possible.

Studying the brain is also difficult because it's so complex. Theoretical physicist Michio Kaku said, "The human brain has 100 billion neurons, each neuron connected to 10,000 other neurons. Sitting on your shoulders is the most complicated object in the known universe."[1] Some scientists call it "the final frontier" in biology because we have understood so little about it.

Medicine has made huge advances in the past hundred years in almost every other area, from healing wounds to treating cancer. We can understand and treat the heart. The liver. The muscles and bones. By comparison, the brain has remained an unknown. The most important factor in our mental and emotional lives is the part of ourselves we know the least about.

Fortunately—slowly but surely—we have finally started making progress.

Scientists have discovered new methods for studying the brain at the very smallest level, the level of individual cells and their even smaller internal parts and pathways. They know more about the molecules that drive brain processes and the barriers that protect the brain from diseases. They've started to understand how damage and disease affect the brain not only in the moment, but over the course of a lifetime.

One of the most important insights from all this new science is that brain health and mental health aren't separate. Brain health *is* mental health. Inflammation is key to both.

---

1   Alison Ebbage, "Thinking Outside the Box: How Does the Brain Work? It Is the Most Complex Computer in the Known Universe yet Its Secrets Have Remained Elusive and Fascinating. Now Techniques Are Being Developed That Are Helping Us to Unravel Its Mysteries," *Engineering & Technology* 15, no. 2 (March 2020): 68–71, https://doi.org/10.1049/et.2020.0210.

WHY DIDN'T ANYONE TELL ME?

When I first went to the doctor to find out why I wasn't getting any better, I didn't hear about any of this. And even when I went out on my own and tried new approaches and they *worked*, my doctors had usually never even heard of them.

While it's true that the brain can be hard to study, and progress in understanding brain health was slow for a long time, there's also another reason doctors sometimes don't, or can't, tell you about the newest information and treatment options: they don't know.

The reasons they don't know are complicated. Many medical professionals are incredibly burnt out from long hours and over-packed schedules. One survey found that 80 percent of doctors reported being at or over their capacity. On top of that, imagine if new information came out every single day on the dozens of diseases and conditions you're in charge of treating. There'd be no way at all to keep up with it all.

Add to that the fact that insurance won't cover a lot of these so-called "alternative" approaches and that doctors are understandably cautious about anything they might prescribe to their patients, and you've got a recipe for slow change at best.

That's why you need to do your own research—which is why you're here, reading this book!

THE LINK TO MENTAL HEALTH

When we talk about mental health, we tend to talk about emotions and feelings. We talk about being depressed or anxious. We use metaphors like "brain fog" or describe symptoms like worry and rumination.

What we usually *don't* do is talk about the brain. When you're depressed, you might say that you feel down, or have dark thoughts, or feel blue, rather than saying, "I have brain problems."

This is kind of odd, when you think about it. If you break your leg, you don't say, "My leg feels unhappy," or "I'm having trouble managing my leg." It's obvious that the problem is a physical one, located in a body part.

The connection between brain health and mental health is a bit less obvious, but just as important.

Modern research has shown that a major factor in mental health conditions and symptoms is the physical health of the brain—or, more accurately, mental health symptoms occur when your brain is in an *unhealthy* state. A state of inflammation.

It turns out almost two-thirds of people experiencing depression and anxiety have higher levels of inflammation. So does almost everyone with sleep issues.[2] And half of those with PTSD.[3] Inflammation is also associated with brain fog, chronic fatigue, long COVID-19, ADHD, schizophrenia, bipolar disorder, autism spectrum disorders, Alzheimer's disease, Parkinson's disease, and diabetes.

You get the idea.

Every single experience you have is at least partly a brain experience. If you get a sunburn from sitting out on the beach for too long, the pain and itching are actually signals your brain is sending in response to sensory input from your skin. If you cry during a romantic movie, that's your brain releasing emotion-producing chemicals into your bloodstream in response to what you see.

2   Paul R. Albert, Chawki Benkelfat, and Laurent Descarries, "The Neurobiology of Depression—Revisiting the Serotonin Hypothesis. I. Cellular and Molecular Mechanisms," *Philosophical Transactions of the Royal Society B* 367, no. 1601 (September 5, 2012): 2378–81, https://doi.org/10.1098/rstb.2012.0190; Christos Pitsavos et al., "Anxiety in Relation to Inflammation and Coagulation Markers, among Healthy Adults: The ATTICA Study," *Atherosclerosis* 185, no. 2 (April 2006): 320–26, https://doi.org/10.1016/j.atherosclerosis.2005.06.001; and Michael R. Irwin, Richard Olmstead, and Judith E. Carroll, "Sleep Disturbance, Sleep Duration, and Inflammation: A Systematic Review and Meta-Analysis of Cohort Studies and Experimental Sleep Deprivation," *Biological Psychiatry* 80, no. 1 (July 1, 2016): 40–52, https://doi.org/10.1016/j.biopsych.2015.05.014.

3   Hiroaki Hori and Yoshiharu Kim, "Inflammation and Post-Traumatic Stress Disorder," *Psychiatry and Clinical Neurosciences* 73, no. 4 (April 2019): 143–53, https://doi.org/10.1111/pcn.12820.

In the same way, if you experience anxiety every time you hear a loud sound, it's not just your ears that are responding. Your brain is telling your body how to feel about that sound and how to react to it. That's why two friends can sit outside at a café, and one of them can be totally overwhelmed by all the people and noise and activity, while the other barely notices. Their brains are interpreting the same situation in different ways.

The same is true with other kinds of mental health issues. The physical health of your brain strongly influences its reactions to experiences. In some cases, physical problems like inflammation can cause your brain to get into a loop and keep reacting long after the original stimulus is gone.

The patterns of how your particular brain interprets and responds to experiences can show up as mental health problems like depression, anxiety, and fatigue. Physical damage to the brain, like what happens with inflammation, can lead to changes in how it interprets and responds. What we call mental health symptoms are often the outward signs of that damage.

WHEN THE BRAIN GOES UNTREATED

It's important to understand the role of the brain in mental health because you can only fix a problem by treating the underlying cause. For example, if you tried to treat a broken leg by popping ibuprofen, you might reduce the pain—but the leg would still be broken. If you never treated the bone itself, it could heal wrong. The pain would get worse.

Then, over decades, the problem could grow and grow, creating other issues like hip and ankle pain. The effects could spread outward through your whole body. You could develop bad posture. That might lead to tension headaches. Constant low-level pain could cause irritability. Eventually, you would have symptoms that seemed totally unrelated to the broken leg.

That's what happens with brain inflammation (also called *neuroinflammation*) and mental health.

When a person has a mental health issue like depression or anxiety, we treat the symptoms. But because we haven't understood the real causes, we rarely treat the underlying problem, which is in the brain.

Over decades, the problem grows. The effects spread outward. There start to be symptoms that seem unrelated to the original cause, the "lightning strike" that started the inflammation in the first place. And even when the original cause is fully treated, the resulting inflammation and its long-term effects can remain.

Once a chronic inflammation cycle has started, your brain acts like an untreated broken leg. The symptoms get worse, and they're harder and harder to trace to the original event. Decades later, you could develop an attention disorder or mental health issues, or any number of other problems, and have no idea that they were caused by that initial "broken leg" of stress or trauma.

Don't worry if you don't get all of this right now. I'll give you a crash course in inflammation science in Chapters Two and Three. That's where you'll learn everything you need to know about how your body uses inflammation to fight disease and cure injury—and how that process can go terribly wrong.

The key thing to remember is this: when your leg is broken, once you finally set the leg, the rest of you can begin to heal. The same is true with chronic inflammation.

In fact, you don't even have to completely eliminate the inflammation to start healing. Just reducing or interrupting the chronic inflammation cycle lets your body begin to recover on its own.

It is possible to come back, even from long-term inflammation damage. But first you need to recognize that it's happening.

NO TWO ALIKE

As I said earlier, chronic brain inflammation never looks exactly the same in different people. My experience with a concussion looks totally different from Ash's chronic work stress, which looks totally different from Stephanie's persistent anxiety and stomach issues.

If they are all impacted by the same underlying problem, why don't they look more alike?

Because humans are incredibly complex. Beyond complex.

Your brain alone has almost as many neurons, or brain cells, as there are stars in the entire Milky Way galaxy.

Your body contains more than thirty *trillion* cells. And every single cell communicates with all the others nearby. Each cell has its own jobs—its own activities and behaviors. And at the same time, every cell is acting on, and interacting with, other cells, creating a new environment in your body with every passing moment.

Over the course of a lifetime, these interactions build and build on each other. Every human body becomes its own totally unique system, unlike any other human body in the world.

Imagine building a series of houses. You might get ten people together and hand them wood beams, nails, bricks, and roofing tiles. Then, down the street, you would get ten different people together to build another house. And on the next block, another group would be building a third house. All the groups would have the same building materials. They would all know, basically, what a house is supposed to look like. But every group's house would end up looking different because the groups would make different decisions along the way.

That's what happens in your body. We're all made up of the same building blocks, like cells and blood vessels and chemicals, but there are tons of complex processes going on all the time. Only instead of ten builders, your body has *trillions* of cells.

Every time the builders made a decision about their house, it would become a little different from all the others. Similarly, every tiny change in your body, even in a single cell, causes you to be a little bit more different from every other human. Over time, these small differences add up. It's no wonder that something like inflammation shows up differently in every person's body.

Add to that the fact that we all start out with different genetics and grow up in different environments, and it's kind of amazing that our reactions to something complex like inflammation have anything in common at all.

Fortunately, they do. What's essentially the same in every human body is the inflammation process itself. The effects, or symptoms, of your chronic brain inflammation might look completely different from mine. In fact, they almost certainly will. But because they have the same underlying problem, it's possible to treat them with similar approaches.

That's what this book is about.

THE MISSING PIECE

When you go to a doctor with a mental health issue, you're usually given two options: medication and therapy. These are tried-and-true approaches, and most doctors are familiar with them. But if your real problem is chronic brain inflammation, they're often not enough on their own.

Medications, for example, can be very effective, but not every person, or every brain, responds the same way. The same medication can have incredibly positive effects for one person, do nothing at all for another, and cause terrible side effects for someone else. It's very difficult to know ahead of time who will benefit and who will have side effects.

Also, most medications are aimed at symptoms. Symptoms are the end result of a problem, not the cause. A medication could work well to control one aspect of your condition, but if it doesn't fix the underlying problem, you'll never get all the way better. Plus, the side effects tend to add up. If you have to take a different medication for every single one of your symptoms, the "cure" can be worse than the disease.

Therapy has the opposite problem. Amazingly enough, therapy can actually help reduce brain inflammation. Researchers are only just learning why and how this works. But it can take months or even years for therapy to address and relieve the problem, and many people need relief now.

The problem is, reducing the underlying inflammation through therapy can take a long time. Even with the best therapist and the most up-to-date approaches, the process can take months or even years to have an effect.

When you're suffering, even a few months can be too long to wait.

Now, don't get me wrong. I am not saying that medication and therapy can't work. They *do* work for some people, and we'll discuss how to choose the best therapy option for your symptoms, if that's what you want, in Section Two.

The missing piece of the traditional treatment puzzle is brain health. The fitness, or health, of your brain creates the lens through which you experience and engage with the world. Your brain creates your entire experience of life, from pain and fatigue to joy and learning.

The brain is an organ just like your liver or your heart. The health of your brain is just as important as the health of any other organ.

The approaches in this book give you the power to improve your brain health directly and improve your quality of life.

This book will introduce you to a lot of different treatment tools and methods. Some of them are simple and can be done at home. Some are based on traditional healing practices that have been validated by modern science. Others are absolutely cutting edge and use brand-new health technologies.

Every approach in this book has been proven by research to improve brain health directly. And I've used a lot of them on myself or with clients working to improve brain inflammation–related problems.

All of them are tools for your brain-health toolbox.

Because they're tools, you don't have to choose just one, and you don't have to use all of them. Your healing might come from a combination of several. In fact, that's very likely. Conventional tools like medication and therapy can be effective in your healing. Medication can reduce symptoms while you fix the underlying inflammation. Therapy can work together with other brain-health treatments to heal the mind and body together.

No matter what your best combination turns out to be, the first step to knowing how to fix the problem is to understand it.

A FRIENDLY CAUTION

The information in this book isn't intended to replace an ongoing relationship with your primary doctor. If you ever notice any significant changes in your health, or have any concerns, your doctor should be the first person you talk to.

In the next two chapters, I'll be leading you on a guided tour of the basics of brain health, inflammation, and stress. I'll show you how inflammation processes that are supposed to heal you can end up hurting you instead. Most importantly, I'll show you why brain health is the basis for everything that is happening to you and the key to overcoming the challenges you're facing.

We'll start by asking ourselves one critically important question: If inflammation causes so much harm, why do we have it at all?

TL;DR

→ If your mental health is suffering, *inflammation* might be the missing piece that explains what is going on with you.

→ When inflammation gets out of control, it can lead to a wide variety of mental health issues and symptoms, especially if it's inflammation in the brain (or *neuroinflammation*).

→ Because it can cause so many different effects, inflammation looks different, or shows up differently, in different people.

→ New science is giving us important insights into the effects of inflammation—and how to deal with it.

CHAPTER TWO

———

HEALING HEAT

The Science of Inflammation

Jadyn realizes he's been staring at the same question for nearly 20 minutes. He was supposed to have finished his coding homework an hour ago, and he's barely halfway through. It's like all of a sudden he can't concentrate. He can't think. He can't remember what he was reading five minutes ago or what he learned from the last video.

And it's not just the homework. At work today, he messed up three coffee orders in a row. He used to be able to hold three, four, even five orders in his head at once. Recently, if he tries to make more than one at a time, he puts in the wrong milks or forgets which ones should be iced or hot. It's embarrassing. His boss nearly lost it today when he had to throw out more than one drink and a customer complained.

The weirdest part, though, is his energy. He's never even thought about energy before because he's always been the life of the party, always up for late nights or road trips or whatever. Now, he finds himself passing out on the couch after work and waking up hours later, still exhausted.

It's starting to make him feel really anxious. Is he going to lose his job? How will he pay for his coding classes? He's going to turn 30 soon, and he really wanted to have a new job by then. Everything was lining up perfectly! And now this.

He wonders whether these new problems have anything to do with COVID. He's young and healthy, so it didn't seem like a big deal when he got it. He was short of breath for a few days, laid out with a bad cough. He missed a week of work, but no big deal.

Two weeks after that, long after he was sure he'd recovered, he started having these weird symptoms. Brain fog that keeps him from studying. Fatigue that seems to physically shove him down onto the couch as soon as he walks through the door. An inability to focus or remember things at work.

And now this week, as if that weren't enough, he's started getting dizzy. Just randomly. He'll be standing in front of the espresso machine at work or jumping up to grab a study snack, and suddenly he'll find himself feeling woozy, with a swirling off-balance sensation in his head.

In those moments, he's really afraid. What's happening to him? Will it last forever? He's too young for this!

Jadyn gives in to his exhaustion and decides he can do the rest of his homework in the morning. He's just too tired. He drags himself to bed, desperately hoping that all this clears up before his big exam next week.

Like a lot of my clients, I met Jadyn at a low moment in his life. He had been a multisport athlete in high school. A friendly, outgoing guy who seemed to never get sick. Until now.

It had been more than three months since his COVID-19 infection, and he wasn't just not recovering. Somehow, he was getting worse.

What Jadyn was experiencing was his immune system in overdrive.

THE CASTLE GUARD

The immune system exists to protect your body from harm. It's a lot like a castle guard.

Think of the last time you saw a movie with castles, guards, and invading forces. I'm a big fan of *Lord of the Rings* and *Shrek* myself. Whatever your favorite version, I'm sure you can picture that moment when an invading army rides up to a castle, only to be stopped by the castle wall. Heavy stone stands between the invaders and the inside of the castle. The drawbridge is drawn up and there is a moat, deep and full of water.

Your body's wall and moat are your skin and mucous membranes (like in your nose and mouth). They're the first line of defense against bacteria, viruses, dirt, and all the other attackers waiting to make you sick or damage your body. You've also got additional protectors like eyelashes, which capture big invaders before they can get into your sensitive eyes. The entire outside of your body is designed to turn away bad guys before they can hurt you.

A lot of potential invaders are stopped right there, never getting any farther.

As effective as it is, though, your skin isn't enough to fight every possible invader. A lot of potentially harmful things get into your body anyway. That's where your immune system comes into play.

Think about an army laying siege to a castle. For hours or days, they are stuck outside the thick castle walls, just trying to get through. But if they are successful, they eventually breach the wall. A battering ram crashes through the main gate or an explosion destroys a portion of the wall itself.

However they manage it, once they are inside, they can do far more damage than they could from outside the wall. Additional defenders are needed. A trumpet rings out as soldiers are called from all different areas of the castle to take on the invading force. All the noise and activity of the battle becomes concentrated at that one spot.

When an invader like bacteria or a virus gets past your skin and outer defenses, your immune system acts as the castle guard. First, your body recognizes something that shouldn't be there. Cells in the injured or damaged area send out distress signals, calling for help. The immune system responds, sending special cells to the damaged areas to fight the invaders, clean up the mess, and hopefully return things to normal.

We'll come back to the castle again soon. But for now, let's zoom in on exactly how the immune system works in your body.

OUCH! IMMUNE SYSTEM TO THE RESCUE

There you are, on a normal Thursday evening, making dinner and thinking about your day.

Oops! Maybe you were thinking about your day more than you were thinking about making dinner. The knife slips, and you cut your finger. It's not deep, but it's bleeding, so you wash it in the sink. The bleeding doesn't stop right away, so you rummage around in the bathroom cabinet and find something to bandage the wound.

You go back to making dinner and don't think much more about it.

But what's going on underneath that bandage? Hidden away under that plastic strip, fascinating processes are taking place. Over the next few days, the cut will heal itself and then disappear. How is that possible?

Right away, as soon as you cut yourself, your body is already performing amazingly complex activities to repair the damage. A special kind of cell (called *platelets*) rushes to the scene of the cut. These cells stick together to form a clot, the first step to stop the bleeding.

These special cells also act like the trumpeter in the castle. They raise the alarm, sending out signals to the immune system. They're basically calling out, "Help! Help! Damage in the left index finger! Calling all immune system responders!"

These signals are sent using so-called "signaling proteins." The scientific name for them is cytokines (sigh-toe-kines). Cytokines are fascinating little molecules, but what you need to know is that cytokines are small messengers that tell cells what to do: where to travel within the body to fight invaders, when to divide and make more cells, and so on. They're a little like carrier pigeons, communicating between different outposts in the body.

They're so important to fixing damage in your body that their number can increase by *a thousand times* in response to an infection or other invader.

Cytokines also warn the immune system to start looking for infection. They call out with their signals, saying, "Something bad happened here. There's been a tear in the outer defenses. Look for trespassers!"

In response, the immune system sends its other big guns, the white blood cells. There are lots of kinds of white blood cells. You might have heard of some of them. There are T cells and B cells, macrophages, and natural killer cells, among others. Again, you don't need to memorize these names or what each type of white blood cell actually does.

What's important is that these different kinds of white blood cells rush to the damaged area and start looking around for problems.

In fact, let's stop for a minute and really focus on how amazing white blood cells are.

They are your body's badasses.

Some of them literally *eat* bacteria and viruses and other bad guys so they can't harm you. Some of them dissolve attacking cells in chemicals called *enzymes*. Others act like inspectors, tagging harmful cells as intruders so other cells know to destroy them later.

Some even "fire" proteins at the bad guys, like characters in a video game.

As they eat or dissolve or tag the attackers, white blood cells are also sending more messages back to headquarters. They can call for backup, letting the body know that more response is needed. They can trigger your body to prepare resources for healing.

White blood cells also release different chemicals that get into the bloodstream in the damaged area. Those chemicals attract more blood. The increased blood flow causes redness, heat, and swelling.

What is another name for redness, heat, and swelling? Yep. The immune response, and white blood cells in particular, cause *inflammation*.

This inflammation isn't a bad thing on its own. In fact, it's necessary for immune function. The increased blood flow to the injured area brings repair tools like additional white blood cells to fix the damage, carries infection fighters throughout the body, and removes dead and damaged cells. You need inflammation to fight your battles.

In other words, **inflammation is part of a healthy immune response.** It's absolutely necessary for protecting your body against harm. Without inflammation, your body would have no defense against the literally billions of bacterial cells, viruses, and other attackers that swirl around us all the time.

Inflammation becomes a problem only when it goes into overdrive and doesn't stop. One very common reason for that is stress.

LIONS AND TIGERS AND ANGRY TEXTS: THE STRESS RESPONSE

In the case of the cut finger, the inflammation process is pretty straightforward. You can literally see it happening. You cut yourself. The cut triggers the immune system to respond. Your finger gets red and swollen and painful. After a few days, it heals. Simple.

But inflammation isn't always this visible or straightforward. Surprisingly, a lot of immune system triggers don't come from the outside at all. Some of them come from within your own body or from "invisible" sources like stress or trauma. You don't have to have an infection to cause inflammation.

STRESS IN THE BODY

When we talk about stress, we're usually talking about a feeling. "I feel stressed" means that I'm overworked or overwhelmed. But stress is more than a feeling. It's a set of physical responses in the body that can activate the immune system.

Yeah, that surprises a lot of people, but it's really important to remember. Stress is *physical*.

Plus, if stress continues for a long time, it creates a self-feeding cycle. The stress causes physical responses in your body, which create more stress, which create more physical responses...

You get the idea.

But what exactly *is* stress, anyway?

Talking in biological terms, **stress is anything that negatively impacts your cells' ability to do their jobs.**

Some stress has positive effects. Exercise is a form of stress that breaks down muscle tissue in the short term, but that breakdown is what allows stronger muscles to be built. Negative stress, on the other hand, is stress that damages cells' ability to function and keeps the body from functioning as it should.

Let's break that down.

Every cell in your body has a job. Fingernail cells make a protein that creates a hard shell, protecting your sensitive fingertips. Special cells in your eyes capture light and color. Muscle cells expand and contract to move your body around.

Your body is made up of close to 200 different types of cells, each with their own jobs. And all those cells have to be performing their jobs in order for your body—and brain—to function.

When you get injured, the effect on your cells is visible from the outside. You bleed. You bruise. You get a scar. Maybe you need a cast. Those are signs of your blood cells and skin cells and bone cells being impacted.

When you experience emotional or internal stress, the effects are much less obvious, but they are just as real. In fact, they can be worse. And the trigger can be something surprisingly small and normal.

Just think about the last time you got an angry text.

WHEN IS AN ANGRY TEXT LIKE A TIGER?

When your body experiences stress from an emotional trigger, a lot of things happen at once.

Let's say you've just arrived for your shift at the grocery store. You look at the assignment sheet and find out you're on restocking. Your back doesn't love the idea, but you head to the back of the store to get started. You've had your coffee, and at least restocking doesn't usually involve a lot of customer interaction. Things aren't looking too bad.

A regular morning. No problem. Until you hear the *ping* of your text message, pull your phone out—and see that it's from your boss.

Apparently, the night crew didn't do their job, and your boss is *mad*. She texts you again before you can even respond to the first one. Another second later, there's a third text. You know it's the night team's fault, but she is taking it out on you.

Suddenly, your breathing seems faster. It's shallow. You can feel pinpricks of sweat along your brow and the insides of your palms. You're lightheaded and your mind is racing.

That first text was the trigger, pushing you into the stress response immediately.

I'm getting worked up just telling this story! And I bet you can relate too. We've all experienced that feeling when something upsetting happens, and your body responds like you've just dodged a runaway city bus.

As soon as you become aware of the stressful input, your body releases hormones like cortisol and adrenaline. Cortisol represses any body functions that aren't immediately necessary for life. Every single activity in your body takes energy, so when you're stressed, your body shuts down anything extra that could use the energy you might need to survive. Adrenaline spikes your heart rate and breathing, getting you ready to run from the danger.

That response is called *fight-or-flight* (sometimes also known as the fight/flee/freeze response), and it's your body's physiological reaction to stress. (We'll come back to the science of fight or flight in more detail in Chapter Three.)

The problem is that the human stress response was built into our bodies long before the invention of texting. Before the invention of writing, for that matter. Back when humans lived in the open, alongside tigers and snakes and other life-threatening neighbors, where a life-or-death response to stress made total sense.

If you live near tigers, and you hear a twig snap behind you, you don't want to stop and think. It's much better to leap ten feet and run away, even if you later realize it was only a bird rustling around in the leaves.

Humans don't have a ton of physical adaptations for surviving danger. We don't run very fast. We don't have camouflage. We can't fly. Out on the open plains, early humans were exposed and vulnerable. The life-or-death, fight-or-flight stress response kept us alive in the face of danger.

Unfortunately, stress is also disruptive. It's hard on the body and brain. It can cause lingering physical and psychological effects. There's a reason we say "I'm stressed out" like it's a bad thing.

Even though most of us don't live near tigers anymore, our bodies haven't gotten the message. Technology evolves much, much faster than the human body and brain. These days, a sudden sound is more likely to be the buzz of a text message or the ping of a Slack notification than a tiger.

Our modern lives are also a lot safer than the lives of early humans. We've learned to live in houses to stay warm and to wear shoes to protect our feet from damage. We have stitches to put ourselves back together if we get injured and casts to heal broken bones.

But our bodies still respond to stressful situations almost exactly the way they did when we lived outside and every stray sound could have been a predator. Unfortunately, unlike deer and other prey animals, we rarely have the chance to just "shake it off," which would complete the cycle and push the stress out of our bodies. We hold it in instead, and the stress sticks with us.

Even more than that, our bodies have become conditioned to respond to *abstract* stressors (like money and relationships) the same way we used to respond to tigers. Our nervous systems respond to just the *idea* of a tiger, even if that "tiger" is really an overdraft notice or a negative comment on social media.

MODERN STRESS, ANCIENT STRESS RESPONSE

If your fight-or-flight response helps you leap out of the way of an oncoming car, that's helpful. Your body reacts before you are even aware of it, and you jump back on the sidewalk out of breath, sweating, heart racing but alive. After a few minutes or hours, the stress hormones flush out of your system, and you go on with your day.

But what if you live in a city, and you hear horns blaring and deal with irritable, busy people all day long? It feels like you get used to it. You no longer leap out of the way every time a car swerves or a bike messenger rushes by. Under the surface, though, your body keeps activating the stress response. You may not notice it consciously, but in the modern world of constant noise and movement and activity, your stress centers stay "on" a lot of the time.

Your boss's text is the same thing. You know, in your mind, that an angry text can't kill you. Your body, on the other hand, responds as if the text were a tiger or a speeding car. That's because the part of your brain that controls this response (the amygdala) doesn't do too well with the nuances of context. There's a game of telephone between the input from your eyes and ears, and the response from various parts of your brain. The brain receives the persistent stress messengers and continuously responds.

Early humans might have lived with predators, but the predators didn't stand behind them all day long, breathing down their necks. They weren't surrounded by predators every minute of the day, which meant they had a chance to let go of the stress and reset. For many of us, living in the modern world is like living inside the tiger's den. We experience one stressor after another, all day long. Job stress. Family stress. Social media. Money issues. Notifications. Traffic. Noise. Pollution. Awful neighbors. Travel. Difficult decisions. It's never ending.

OPPRESSION, STRESS, AND INFLAMMATION

There are few things more stressful than experiencing bias or discrimination. Unfortunately, people who live with injustice due to race, socioeconomic status, sexual or gender identity, or culture of origin don't experience just daily acute stressors as a result. These factors are also associated with higher levels of depression, anxiety, and PTSD, as well as chronic inflammation.[4]

Imagine a kid growing up in a neglected neighborhood in an inner city. His parents both dropped out of high school because they had to work to help support their families. His dad works at night, and his mom's shifts at the hospital change every week, so his schedule is chaotic and unpredictable. Plus, he's been the target of kids at school. His parents work really hard to send him to a better school, but that means he has to catch a bus at 6:30 in the morning, and he's one of the only kids of color in the school.

Even if he does well in life, moves to a better neighborhood, has a great career, and raises his own family, he's more likely to experience all kinds of inflammatory issues later in life.

Parents with lower education levels, for example, tend to have higher stress—and as a result, their kids also experience more stress.[5] Children who grow up in these homes often show substantially increased cortisol long afterward, even into adulthood.[6]

---

4 Monnica Williams, Muna Osman, and Chrysalis Hyon, "Understanding the Psychological Impact of Oppression Using the Trauma Symptoms of Discrimination Scale," *Chronic Stress* 7 (January 2023), https://doi.org/10.1177/24705470221149511.

5 Amanda R. Tarullo et al., "Cortisol and Socioeconomic Status in Early Childhood: A Multidimensional Assessment," *Development and Psychopathology* 32, no. 5 (December 2020): 1876–87, https://doi.org/10.1017/s0954579420001315.

6 Amy S. Desantis, Christopher W. Kuzawa, and Emma K. Adam, "Developmental Origins of Flatter Cortisol Rhythms: Socioeconomic Status and Adult Cortisol Activity," *American Journal of Human Biology* 27, no. 4 (July/August 2015): 458–67, https://doi.org/10.1002/ajhb.22668.

Being a member of a racial minority that experiences discrimination can also lead to later-life chronic inflammation and inflammation-related diseases.[7] The same is true for people who are diverse in their sexuality or gender. Their higher levels of health problems in later life have been tied to chronic inflammation resulting from the stress of social threats like rejection, stigma, and isolation.[8]

Any of these factors can also lead to being socially isolated as a kid—which on its own predicts chronic inflammation as much as 40 years later.[9] By the time the kid is old enough to make changes in their own life, the damage is done.[10]

Discrimination isn't just unfortunate. It can be dangerous to your health.

EVERYDAY STRESS ADDS UP

Maybe it seems obvious that living with severe stressors or discrimination can have lifelong effects.

What's not so obvious is that a series of minor stressors can also have a major impact on long-term brain and mental health.

Think back on the last couple of weeks. Were there any days that you would call stressful? I am willing to bet there were. The impacts of those everyday feelings of stress can be far-reaching.

7   Ronald L. Simons et al., "Racial Discrimination, Inflammation, and Chronic Illness among African American Women at Midlife: Support for the Weathering Perspective," *Journal of Racial and Ethnic Health Disparities* 8 (2021): 339–49, https://doi.org/10.1007%2Fs40615-020-00786-8; and Phoebe H. Lam et al., "Race, Socioeconomic Status, and Low-Grade Inflammatory Biomarkers across the Lifecourse: A Pooled Analysis of Seven Studies," *Psychoneuroendocrinology* 123 (January 2021): 104917, https://pubmed.ncbi.nlm.nih.gov/33160231/.

8   Lisa M. Diamond, Adrian J. Dehlin, and Jenna Alley, "Systemic Inflammation as a Driver of Health Disparities among Sexually-Diverse and Gender-Diverse Individuals," *Psychoneuroendocrinology* 129 (July 2021): 105215, https://pubmed.ncbi.nlm.nih.gov/34090051/.

9   Rebecca E. Lacey, Meena Kumari, and Mel Bartley, "Social Isolation in Childhood and Adult Inflammation: Evidence from the National Child Development Study," *Psychoneuroendocrinology* 50 (December 2014): 85–94, https://doi.org/10.1016/j.psyneuen.2014.08.007.

10 Keely A. Muscatell, Samantha N. Brosso, and Kathryn L. Humphreys, "Socioeconomic Status and Inflammation: A Meta-Analysis," *Molecular Psychiatry* 25 (October 19, 2018): 2189–99, https://doi.org/10.1038/s41380-018-0259-2.

One large-scale study recently showed that experiencing *any* stressful event on a given day can make you feel more depressed—and can also make it more difficult to feel positive emotions when good things do happen. Having an argument *and avoiding one* were both considered stressful. (Makes sense, right? Keeping tough feelings inside can be just as painful as the conflict itself.) Everyday difficulties at work or school—even a stressful event happening to a close friend or family member—all had negative effects on mood and emotions.

Nothing new there. Stressful days happen to all of us, and they're hard.

What's incredible is that the study only initially followed these people for *eight days*. Eight days of looking at their ups and downs in response to stress could predict illness and death *up to two decades later.*[11]

I'm not telling you this to make you worry or to make it seem like you're destined to get chronic inflammation and disease. Far from it.

In fact, I'm telling you the opposite.

Using the tools in this book will increase your resilience and your ability to bounce back from everyday stressors. You'll reduce your reactivity, meaning you won't feel as on edge or fearful. All of these shifts can improve your quality of life directly, but they'll also lower your risk for developing chronic inflammation and help you fight the inflammation you already have.

Okay, so I keep saying that stress leads to inflammation. But how exactly does that happen?

STRESS AND INFLAMMATION

Let's take a bird's-eye view for a moment—literally. Imagine that you can float up out of your house, over the city or town or wherever you live. From way up over the streets and houses, you can see the cars moving from place to place, the streets and roads running in all directions.

From this high up, you notice something interesting. Trucks. There

---

11 N. L. Sin et al., "Affective Reactivity to Daily Stressors Is Associated with Elevated Inflammation," *Health Psychology* 34, no. 12 (December 2015): 1154–65, https://psycnet.apa.org/doi/10.1037/hea0000240.

are delivery trucks everywhere. Blue vans rushing orders to waiting customers. Eighteen-wheelers sighing up to loading docks to unload pallets full of supplies. Refrigerated trucks bringing ingredients to restaurants. All these deliveries being made, all over the city, all day and night—each truck dropping its haul and then returning to the warehouse for more.

Essentially, that's what is happening in your body as well.

Your blood vessels are like highways and side streets. Some are big and fast moving. Others are narrower, like back alleys. Through all of them, blood rushes out to every part of your body, delivering nutrients, oxygen, messengers, immune cells, and all the other things your cells need to thrive.

When your body is relaxed and healthy, the blood vessels are wide open. They're like eight-lane highways. Blood cells, nutrients, and chemical messengers tumble and roll through the wide-open vessels at top speed. Deliveries reach every area of the body, from your toenails to your scalp, and from your vital organs to every inch of your brain.

When you experience stress, the fight-or-flight response narrows some blood vessels and dilates (or opens up) others. This allows the body to direct energy, food, and oxygen to the most important places. Your heart rate speeds up so you're ready to sprint, pushing blood around the body faster. Blood is rushed preferentially to the big muscles so you can run faster or fight harder, while it's drawn away from other places, like your stomach, hands, and feet. (After all, if you're about to get eaten, digestion isn't that important!)

More critically, there's also decreased blood flow to the part of the brain (called the *prefrontal cortex*) that's responsible for higher-level thinking, decision-making, and rationalization.

If the stress is acute and over quickly, your body recovers. The blood vessels open back up, and the highways are ready for traffic again. It's like passing a minor accident on the highway. You might get stuck in backed-up traffic for a few minutes, but once you're past the accident, you can move at highway speeds again.

Chronic stress is different. When stress is chronic, some of your blood vessels stay narrowed, like a four-lane highway suddenly stuck with only one lane open for months. Oxygen and nutrients aren't getting to all the cells anymore, at least not at a healthy rate. All the delivery trucks are backed up in a permanent construction zone, and deliveries are few and far between.

When cells don't get what they need, they don't just sit quietly and wait. Some of them die, alerting the body's cleanup systems. Others send out distress signals, calling for help.

Sound familiar? It's just like what happened when you cut your finger. Cells sending out distress signals can only mean one thing: turning on the immune system.

This time, there's no injury or infection. There's no tangible physical cause—just stress. But the result is the same. The immune system is activated. White blood cells and messengers come rushing to the scene.

Result? Inflammation.

When the stressors continue, or pile up, over weeks or months or years, this process becomes a self-feeding cycle. Over time, the inflammation itself causes stress to nearby cells. Those cells call out for help. The immune system is activated again.

Result? More inflammation. And the cycle continues.

Plus, the more strain on your body, the more parts of your body are impacted. Eventually, the inflammation spreads to the very seat of power itself. The hub. The command center.

Your brain.

TROUBLE INSIDE THE CASTLE

Just how important is your brain?

The obvious answer is that the brain plays a role in *everything*, including breathing.

Even though it's only 2 percent of your body's weight, the brain uses up 20 percent of your energy and resources. It's so important that it's the only part of the body with its own protective shell.

Need more evidence? How's this? Your brain is so important that it's *protected from your own body*.

If your body is a castle, your brain is the royal court, the throne room—the great hall. This is where decisions are made. It's where the most important people gather. It's the command center. As a result, this part of the castle is heavily protected.

In movies, if someone tries to get in to see the queen or king, they are stopped by guards with swords. Your brain is the same way. It is protected and kept separate to preserve its ability to function.

If the body gets sick, the brain needs to stay separate so it can coordinate the response without being compromised. It can't afford to get sick when the body needs its input. The brain also has special types of cells and molecules that enable it to function. These cells (including neurons) and molecules (called *neurotransmitters*) allow the brain to process information and send signals, and they can't be allowed to leak out into the body and be diluted.

The brain even has its own separate immune system. That's how important it is to keep it protected from the rest of your body.

That's where the blood-brain barrier comes in.

The blood-brain barrier is a system of defenders and checkpoints. It keeps most things in the blood from getting into the brain and messing up its delicate functions. It also keeps the important brain-specific messengers and cells from getting out.

The blood-brain barrier is so tightly secured that it has actually slowed down the development of drugs for the brain.[12] Even if your body absorbs a particular drug, the blood-brain barrier often keeps it from reaching brain cells.

You know how in movies like *Mission: Impossible*, agents always have to swipe their key cards to get access to top-secret areas? The blood-brain barrier is like that. Any cell or protein or messenger that wants to get into or out of the brain has to show its credentials.

In this case, the credentials are biological signals instead of ID badges or key cards, but it's the same idea. Security is tight.

Although—oddly enough, it's not as tight as we once thought.

---

12 William M. Pardridge, "Drug Transport across the Blood–Brain Barrier," *Journal of Cerebral Blood Flow & Metabolism* 32, no. 11 (November 2012): 1959–72, https://doi.org/10.1038%2Fjcbfm.2012.126.

For a long, long time, scientists thought the brain was totally separated from the body. They thought the blood-brain barrier was unbreachable. It turns out, that's not quite the case.

The blood-brain barrier does keep the brain protected, but there are doors. After all, if no messages got through at all, the brain wouldn't know what was going on in the body. It wouldn't know when to plan a defense or what kind of response to send.

In reality, the blood-brain barrier is more like a filter than a wall. Certain messengers are allowed in. The newest scientific research has shown us that even the body's immune cells can sometimes get past the barrier.[13] That includes white blood cells.[14] No one thought that was possible until very, very recently.

And what do we know about white blood cells? Yep. Where there are white blood cells, there's inflammation.

When the brain itself gets inflamed, the entire response system is compromised. If your hand is injured, it hurts, but it's localized. If your brain is injured or infected, it affects the entire body. Any system the brain is in charge of could suffer. Digestion.[15] Movement.[16] Mood.[17] Sleep.[18] Memory.[19] Energy levels.[20] The immune system itself.

13 Diana Kwon, "Guardians of the Brain: How a Special Immune System Protects Our Grey Matter," *Nature*, June 1, 2022, https://www.nature.com/articles/d41586-022-01502-8.

14 Joost Smolders et al., "Tissue-Resident Memory T Cells Populate the Human Brain," *Nature Communications* 9 (November 2018): 4593, https://doi.org/10.1038/s41467-018-07053-9.

15 Qin Xiang Ng et al., "The Role of Inflammation in Irritable Bowel Syndrome," *Journal of Inflammation Research* 11 (September 21, 2018): 345–49, https://doi.org/10.2147/jir.s174982.

16 Elif Çınar, Banu Cahide Tel, and Gürdal Şahin, "Neuroinflammation in Parkinson's Disease and Its Treatment Opportunities," *Balkan Medical Journal* 39, no. 5 (September 2022): 318–33, https://doi.org/10.4274/balkanmedj.galenos.2022.2022-7-100.

17 Moisés E. Bauer and Antônio L. Teixeira, "Neuroinflammation in Mood Disorders: Role of Regulatory Immune Cells," *Neuroimmunomodulation* 28, no. 3 (August 2021): 99–107, https://doi.org/10.1159/000515594.

18 Mark R. Zielinksi and Allison J. Gibbons, "Neuroinflammation, Sleep, and Circadian Rhythms," *Frontiers in Cellular and Infection Microbiology* 12 (March 2022), https://doi.org/10.3389/fcimb.2022.853096.

19 Elettra Capogna et al., "Associations of Neuroinflammatory IL-6 and IL-8 with Brain Atrophy, Memory Decline, and Core AD Biomarkers—in Cognitively Unimpaired Older Adults," *Brain, Behavior, and Immunity* 113 (October 2023): 56–65, https://doi.org/10.1016/j.bbi.2023.06.027.

20 Henrik Heitmann et al., "Fatigue, Depression, and Pain in Multiple Sclerosis: How Neuroinflammation Translates into Dysfunctional Reward Processing and Anhedonic Symptoms," *Multiple Sclerosis Journal* 28, no. 7 (June 2022): 1020–27, https://doi.org/10.1177/1352458520972279.

Everything is at risk.

What happens when inflammation goes haywire is the subject of Chapter Three. But before we get there, let's check back in with Jadyn. It's been months since he got sick, but he's still getting worse. He doesn't understand what's happening. Could inflammation and the immune response explain his problem?

IT GOT BETTER, SO WHY AM I WORSE?

When Jadyn got COVID-19, his body responded exactly the way it's designed to do.

His immune system dove into action. Chemical messengers were sent. White blood cells rushed to the rescue, disabling and destroying the infection.

But then the infection was gone, and the immune system had healed the damage, except...it didn't turn off correctly. The self-feeding inflammation cycle set in, damaging cells, eventually hurting the brain itself. With his busy schedule, late nights studying, and the daily demands at work, his body and brain didn't have the rest they needed to fully repair, and quiet the inflammation cycle.

In other words, COVID-19 isn't really why Jadyn is feeling fatigued and confused and dizzy. COVID-19 was just the lightning strike that lit the forest fire.

The defenders that were supposed to be keeping Jadyn safe accidentally turned on him. His own immune system is now hurting him, and possibly hurting him worse than the original COVID-19 infection did. It's as if the guards around the castle did a great job fighting off invaders, but once all the invaders were gone, they turned and started fighting each other.

So how, exactly, does inflammation go from defender to attacker? How does it go from friend to foe?

That's what we're about to find out. Camilla, unfortunately, knows firsthand what it's like.

TL;DR

→ The *immune system* is part of your body's built-in defense against stress, injury, and illness. Inflammation is a normal part of that system's functioning.

→ *Stress* is anything that impedes your cells' ability to do their jobs. That can include everything from physical injury to illness, or problems at work or at home.

→ Chronic (long-term) stress can cause the inflammation cycle to turn on...and not turn off again. This results in chronic inflammation and its life-altering symptoms.

→ Even "minor" stressors experienced over time can create an inflammatory effect that can have major impacts, *decades later.*

_____

CHAPTER THREE

FROM FRIEND TO FOE

One of Camilla's earliest memories is being woken roughly in the dead of night. She was only five years old. Her father shook her and said, "Time to go!" And that was it. Her whole life changed.

Her family left their home before dawn. Camilla shouldered her small backpack, holding her mother's hand and not looking back. The streets were quiet. That by itself was strange. There was usually fighting somewhere nearby, but not tonight. She tried to hold back her fear as her parents rushed her through the sleeping city.

Over the next six months, they lived in camps. Sometimes they were in tents with dozens of other families. Sometimes they had space to themselves. They moved constantly from one camp to another. Finally, they arrived in the United States. Their new California apartment was dark and damp, in the basement of someone else's home. But at least there wasn't a war going on outside.

Over time, Camilla almost forgot the six months of terror her family endured as refugees. She was so young. These days, she doesn't spend a lot of time thinking about the camps or the years of poverty.

These days, she has pain.

From the outside, Camilla's life is going well. She has achieved her lifelong dream of becoming a psychotherapist. She spends her days helping others. She is a healer. A listener. After years of practice in a hospital, she has started her own business and sees clients in her home.

But now, just when everything seems to be falling into place, her physical symptoms are getting worse.

It's 9:00 a.m. and today, Camilla's woken up in pain, stiff all over her body, having hardly slept at all. She's crouching over to walk, and it takes nearly ten minutes just to make it to the bathroom. A hot bath and an extra pain pill help just enough so she doesn't have to cancel the morning's clients, but as the day goes on, she thinks that might have been a mistake.

It's not that the symptoms are new. She's lived with this fatigue and pain for years. It's just that recently, it's been getting worse. The symptoms are starting to take over her life. Moving to a one-story home was supposed to help, but it hasn't done as much as she hoped.

She's desperately afraid that, if the pain and fatigue get any worse, she's going to have to give up her work. She doesn't know what her life will be like without her clients and her profession. So she puts on her "I'm fine" mask and meets with clients and pushes herself through the day. She falls into bed that night in pure exhaustion, only to find that, yet again, she can't sleep.

Once in a while it occurs to her that, just maybe, her early childhood trauma might have something to do with these symptoms. But how could that be? How could being a refugee at five years old cause pain and fatigue in her 40s? She pushes the thought aside. It must just be aging. Or early menopause. Right?

A BROKEN THERMOSTAT

Chronic inflammation is like a broken thermostat. The heat goes up and up and up and never turns off.

When the thermostat in your home is working properly, it's an important part of your comfort and safety. It keeps your home the right temperature for your health and well-being. You can work and make dinner and do all the other things you need to do, without having to think about whether the pipes will freeze.

If your thermostat gets damaged, though, it can wreak havoc.

It's like the time a friend of mine went on vacation to escape the Pacific Northwest winter and left a window cracked in her house. Unfortunately, it was the window right next to the thermostat in her living room. Cold air seeped in through the opening all day and night. The thermostat, sensing the cold temperature, did what it's designed to do. It kept the heater running.

And running. And running. And running.

The temperature on the thermostat itself, next to the open window, kept reading 61 degrees. But in the rest of the house, the rooms were getting warmer and warmer. By the time my friend got back from vacation two weeks later, the house was like an oven. Her houseplants were dead or dying. The chocolate in the bag on the counter was melted together into a clump. More importantly, her furnace was making terrifying noises from being overworked for so long.

Camilla's body is like a house with a broken thermostat. When she experienced trauma as a child, her stress response kicked on. Fight-or-flight reactions amped up. Her immune system launched into overdrive and never fully turned off. Inflammation that started decades ago has been spreading throughout her body and brain ever since, causing an increasing burden of symptoms that combined to make it hard to get through the day—but don't feel related to each other.

The link between chronic inflammation and these kinds of mental and physical burdens is so new that even Camilla, a trained psychotherapist, is not aware of it.

In this chapter, I'm going to show you what happens when your body's thermostat is broken. The breakdown can happen over time from long-term stress, or it can happen all at once as a result of a single traumatic event. Either way, if the inflammation isn't treated, the short-term effects can become long-term symptoms.

The whole thing starts with balance. Your thermostat is designed to keep your home a comfortable, even temperature. Your body is the same way. It needs to maintain a balance between all its different processes, molecules, and parts in order to stay healthy.

The balance in your body is called *homeostasis*, and without it, things can get out of whack very quickly.

KEEPING AN EVEN KEEL

Homeostasis comes from the Greek words for "the same" and "steady."

You need to stay steady inside because the world outside doesn't.

If you go outside in the summer, suddenly you're in the heat. You go into an over–air conditioned bank, and now it's freezing. You go for a walk or a run, and your heartbeat and breathing speed up. Your child starts screaming in the night, and you are out of bed and responding before you realize it.

Despite everything that's happening around you, your body needs to maintain balance. It needs a steady internal temperature to run properly. Cells need to keep getting fuel no matter what you're doing. Your muscles need to keep working, and your brain has to stay online. **All of the processes that run inside your body require a steady, predictable environment to continue working.**

That's why you sweat when it's hot out. Your body temperature increases, and to counter that, your body releases water onto the skin. The water evaporates, cooling you down.

On the flip side, it's also why high fevers are dangerous. If your body gets too far outside its desired steady internal temperature, critical functions start breaking down.

Homeostasis isn't just about temperature though. Every single process inside your body works within a narrow range of inputs. If certain hormones are too low or too high, you won't have enough energy to get through the day or be able to stay asleep at night.

Your body has lots of tools to stay in homeostasis. Like an operator at a switchboard, or a DJ with a sound mixer, the body can increase response in one area, decrease it in another, and so on—all to keep the system in balance.

One of the most important tools for staying in homeostasis is something called *allostasis*.

If homeostasis is the "even keel" your body likes to stay inside of, allostasis is how it deals with *not* being in an even keel all the time. Basically, allostasis means "stability through change."

Why does this matter? Because allostasis is how your body gets used to new stuff. How it adapts to and positively changes your homeostasis.

Take exercise, for example.

Exercise wreaks havoc on your homeostasis. You get hot and sweaty. Your breathing increases. Your muscles work, burning fuel. You expend a bunch of energy.

If your body likes to stay the same, how does it cope? It copes through allostasis. Think about how you feel the first time you exercise after a long time away. You take a long walk, and when you get to those long stairs at the other end of the park, you find yourself huffing and puffing, and you're out of breath and have to stop and rest by the time you get to the top.

But if you take that same walk again later in the week, and keep it up over time, it gets easier. Your lungs and heart handle it better. A few weeks later, you realize you've made it up those stairs without stopping, and you're not really even breathing hard.

What's happened here is that you've *adapted* to the stress of exercise. Your body's homeostasis range has expanded and can handle more than it used to. That's what allostasis makes possible: it's a response to stress that allows us to grow.

In fact, that's one of the big benefits of exercise: expanding your body's ability to respond to physical stress.

If you've ever planted vegetable seeds, you know how this works. Being from the Pacific Northwest, I can tell you that it stays cold pretty late in the year. If you put the seeds in the ground too early, they'll freeze and die. But if you wait to plant them when it's nice and warm, you won't get many vegetables before they start to fade in the summer heat.

So you expose them to the cold a little at a time. You plant the seeds in cups and leave them in the kitchen. Then you move them to a cold window, then maybe out to the shed. If you do it right, the plants adapt, and you can go ahead and plant them when it's colder than they normally like.

In other words, thank goodness for allostasis. If homeostasis keeps us within the healthy range, allostasis expands the range we can experience as healthy.

That's especially important when it comes to handling stress.

Despite how we talk about it, stress isn't all bad. Going for a run is stressful. Going to college is stressful. These things push us, but thanks to allostasis, we can adapt—as long as the stress stays within our adaptable range.

It's when stress gets away from us, pushed beyond what we can handle (especially if that goes on for a long time) that we can get into trouble. The overall amount of stress you've handled in your life is known as your *allostatic load*. It's a measure of how much you've had to adapt. A higher allostatic load is associated with all kinds of poor physical and mental health outcomes.[21]

If stress drives us to change, adapt, and respond, then how exactly does that happen in the body? Let's take a look under the hood.

STRESS RESPONSE SQUAD: TEAM SAM AND TEAM HPA

The first job of the stress response is to get you the heck away from danger. That's so important that your body isn't really concerned with the damage or disruption it's sustaining.

It's the same reason firefighters carry axes as well as hoses. When

---

21 Jenny Guidi et al., "Allostatic Load and Its Impact on Health: A Systematic Review," *Psychotherapy and Psychosomatics* 90, no. 1 (December 2020): 11–27, https://doi.org/10.1159/000510696.

your house is on fire, there's no time to worry about whether they're damaging your walls. They need to get to the source of the flame and evacuate everyone inside, *now*.

At that point, they bring in the water, cooling down the temperature and dousing the fire. Evacuating people prevents immediate injury and harm, but it doesn't solve the underlying problem, which is the fire. Unfortunately, putting out the fire can also wreak utter havoc to your home—sometimes even more than the fire itself.

In your body, your responders are the SAM system and the HPA axis. We'll call them Team SAM and Team HPA. Team SAM are the first responders, rushing in to save you from danger, disrupting the system in order to save it. Team HPA works more gradually, flooding your system with what you need to survive the stress.

Both Team SAM and Team HPA are necessary for you to respond to, and survive, stressors. Both, and especially Team HPA, are also necessary to keep your body in balance (or get it back into balance after a disruption). And both, unfortunately, can also drive inflammation and damage in your body.

Let's look at them a little closer.

NEED-TO-KNOW, OR NEAT TO KNOW?

A quick word before we dive deep into the science of the SAM system and the HPA axis. These are complex systems. The science can be hard to understand, with lots of new terminology and complicated relationships.

Don't let that worry you. The last thing I want to do is stress you out (obviously!).

If you don't remember every technical term in this section, that won't hurt your ability to benefit from the powerful inflammation-busting approaches in the rest of the book. This information is here to help you understand what's going on in your body when you experience stress and how that leads to long-term problems.

There are really only two critical points to remember. First: the SAM system is your body's "first responder" to stress, while the HPA axis takes longer to respond. Second, the HPA axis is central to keeping your body in balance—and you need that balance to stay healthy in body and mind.

Everything else in this section is on a neat-to-know basis.

THE SAM SYSTEM

When you experience a stressor, Team SAM responds immediately, within seconds. SAM basically lights up the board and yells, "This is an emergency! All systems go!"

The SAM's primary role is to activate adrenaline.

SAM stands for sympathetic-adrenal-medullary pathway. In other words, the SAM system is turned on by the *sympathetic nervous system* (S), which activates a part of the adrenal gland called the *adrenal medulla* (AM). This is a fancy way of saying the job of the SAM is to activate adrenaline.

Adrenaline is what you feel when you get scared or excited. It puts your body on high alert, raising your blood pressure and increasing your heart rate. If you need to leap to pull your child's hand away from a hot stove, you should thank your adrenal glands! On the other hand, if you have a micromanaging boss who's always popping into your office out of nowhere, your constantly raised heart rate and nervous sweating are also the result of adrenaline.

When that happens, adrenaline (made by the adrenal glands) rushes into the bloodstream, kicking on all the fight-or-flight symptoms: elevated heart rate and breathing, increased blood pressure, pupil dilation...all the stuff that gets you ready to fight or run away.

The SAM system gets the fast-acting, immediate stress response going, letting you respond to danger within seconds.

THE HPA AXIS

The HPA axis is the other part of the stress-response system. It's slower-acting but longer-lasting, and it also plays a key role in managing homeostasis in your body. It's a little more complicated than the SAM system, too, so we'll go through it in a bit more detail.

The letters "HPA" stand for hypothalamus, pituitary gland, and adrenal glands. So what does that mean?

Short version: while SAM acts really quickly by releasing adrenaline to give you an immediate burst of energy, the HPA axis uses hormones to help your body respond over a longer time.

The longer version looks like this:

The *hypothalamus* is a structure in your brain. It's deep down in the very center of the brain, and it acts as the link between your brain and your hormones. Your hormones are messengers that travel around in your bloodstream and tell your cells and organs what to do. For example, if you eat food, there are hormones that tell your stomach to start digesting the food. If you run, other hormones tell your body to sweat. But how do the hormones themselves know what to do? How does your body know when to release a hormone or stop releasing one? The hypothalamus tells them.

The *pituitary gland* is located at the base of the hypothalamus. A gland is an organ that makes the substances your body needs. When the brain decides that a hormone is needed, it tells one of your glands to manufacture it and release it into the blood. The pituitary gland is known as the "master gland" because it controls other glands in your hormone system. The pituitary gland is important in your stress response because it releases, or tells other glands to release, all the messengers that amp up your body for fight-or-flight.

Which takes us to the adrenal glands.

Like the SAM system, the HPA axis also activates the *adrenal glands*. Located near the kidneys, just below your rib cage at the back of your body, the adrenal glands produce a number of stress-related hormones, including cortisol and adrenaline.

It can look like the SAM system and the HPA axis are doing the same thing, but the slower HPA response is important because it maintains a more even level of hormones over time than the quick-release of the SAM system. Also, the hormones released by the HPA axis trigger other responses. For example, the HPA axis can prompt your liver and your fat cells to release stored energy, giving you the boost you need to outrun that tiger—or make it through your annual performance review.

STRESS AND HPA IMBALANCE

The point here isn't to memorize what "HPA" stands for or to remember all the specific processes or terminology.

The point is that the HPA axis is key in maintaining balance and homeostasis in your body.

The fight-or-flight response disrupts the normal working of the HPA axis. When you're not stressed, the HPA axis maintains the balance between your nervous system, your hormone (endocrine) system, and your immune system. Even momentary fight-or-flight activations can push it out of whack, but when you're healthy, it bounces back pretty quickly.

When you deal with constant or repeated stress, or live in a stressful situation you can't escape from, that continual HPA axis activation pushes all three systems out of balance, creating longer-term symptoms and creating a feedback loop. The imbalance causes more stress, which causes more imbalance, and so on.

Whatever your symptoms, if you have chronic inflammation, you probably have some kind of imbalance in the HPA axis. That means any treatment plan you choose has to do more than treat symptoms. It has to get the HPA axis back in balance—or at least get close enough to turn down the chronic inflammation cycle and let your body heal.

One of the most crucial tasks of adulthood is to make decisions. Sometimes you have days or months to think about them, and sometimes you have to decide yes or no right now, especially in an emergency. Either way, good decisions require the ability to use objective information to decide on the best course of action.

Childhood trauma can damage that ability.

Many people who have suffered childhood abuse and neglect struggle with something called *impulsivity*—not just during childhood but into adolescence and adulthood.[22] Impulsivity means acting without thought, especially without thought about the consequences. It can lead to risky behaviors like quitting jobs or engaging in high-risk sex, creating severe havoc in a person's life.

Childhood traumatic experiences can also lead to difficulty assessing the real danger of a situation. Adults who have suffered trauma early in life often feel anxiety when there is nothing objectively anxiety-causing in their environment. As a result, they tend to overlook objective information like context and instead respond quickly, impulsively, and inaccurately—on the basis of fear rather than information.[23]

To learn more about childhood trauma and its causes and effects, check out Bessel van der Kolk's book *The Body Keeps the Score.*

The impact of childhood trauma on the people who have lived through it is just starting to be fully understood. But it doesn't have to be irreversible.

---

22 David F. Marshall et al., "Deficient Inhibitory Control as an Outcome of Childhood Trauma," *Psychiatry Research* 235 (January 30, 2016): 7–12, https://doi.org/10.1016/j.psychres.2015.12.013; and Sunny H. Shin, Shelby Elaine McDonald, and David Conley, "Profiles of Adverse Childhood Experiences and Impulsivity," *Child Abuse & Neglect* 85 (November 2018): 118–26, https://doi.org/10.1016/j.chiabu.2018.07.028.

23 Laura Castañón, "Childhood Trauma Changes Your Brain. But It Doesn't Have to be Permanent," *Northeastern Global News*, February 20, 2020, https://news.northeastern.edu/2020/02/20/childhood-trauma-changes-your-brain-but-it-doesnt-have-to-be-permanent/.

THE DOMINO EFFECT

Stressors that don't get turned off cause all sorts of problems. From thyroid disease to fatigue to sleep issues, an imbalanced HPA axis affects every major system in the body. Imbalance in the HPA axis can even turn the immune system against your own healthy cells, causing autoimmune disorders.[24]

Let's call it the domino effect.

Basically, when one thing goes wrong, it triggers other things to go wrong, which trigger other things, and so on.

Let's go back to our friends the firefighters, arriving at the scene of an apartment fire.

Except—unfortunately—the firefighters themselves are stuck behind an accident three blocks away, so the first responders to arrive are the paramedics. They pull up, lights and sirens blaring, and then they have to...wait.

They can't go inside because the fire is still blazing out of control. They don't know whether anyone's injured because they can't go inside. So they pull up in front of the house and hold.

Finally, the fire engine shows up! It screeches into the cul-de-sac, only to find that the ambulance is parked in front of the apartment building already. The paramedics rush to move their vehicle, only to get blocked in when the fire chief arrives in his SUV.

It takes precious minutes to untangle that mess, but then the engine is set up, and...where is the ladder truck? It's stuck in the same traffic the engine was stuck in. And since the fire is on the fourth floor, they need that ladder.

And all this time, the paramedics are waiting and can't report the incident to the hospital because they don't know whether there are any injuries. So the hospital can't prepare the right medical response either.

Meanwhile, the fire is spreading. What started as a kitchen fire

---

24 Marcello Bagnasco, Irene Bossert, and Giampaolo Pesce, "Stress and Autoimmune Thyroid Diseases," *Neuroimmunomodulation* 13, no. 5–6 (August 2007): 309–317, https://doi.org/10.1159/000104859.

in a single apartment is becoming a major incident across several floors of the building.

What would normally be a minor inconvenience—a slight traffic delay—has turned into a major crisis as one problem caused another, which caused another, the domino effect in action.

In the same way, your body's response to stress isn't just one thing. It's a complex coordination between multiple different systems, communicating along multiple channels and operating in finely tuned balance. Allostasis makes you resilient enough to rebound from most minor incidents. But like the fire responders, if you're hit with one thing after another, or if the stress response is turned on and never turned off, the problems start to compound.

Every step out of balance causes other systems to speed up or slow down to compensate. Over time, the situation grows and grows. What was once a small or one-time problem now has the whole system in overdrive, trying to catch up. Every system that shifts to catch up causes more imbalance, shifting others, keeping the cycle going.

That's what happened to Camilla. She was hit, hard, by a major stressor in childhood: the trauma of being a refugee. But then, even when she was safe, she found her family living in poverty. Another stressor—and one she couldn't escape from.

Over time, her symptoms got worse. The cycle turned on and didn't turn off. And now, decades later, she is still feeling the effects.

The domino effect of chronic stress can be tipped off by any number of experiences or events in your life. But in general, there are two types of experiences that cause it. They're called *persistent stressors* and *traumatic events*, and they're what we're going to talk about next.

MORE THAN ONE TYPE OF STRESS

Stress can show up in our lives in a lot of different ways. Stress can refer to severe, short-lived experiences or to long, drawn-out problems that affect our lives for a long time. These are generally known as *acute stress* and *chronic stress*.

Persistent stressors are a form of chronic stress, whereas traumatic events are acute.

Acute stress is immediate, powerful, and over quickly. Stubbing your toe is an acute stressor. Jumping out of the way of a speeding bike messenger is an acute stressor. Getting laid off is an acute stressor. So is a seasonal flu. Your body is designed to respond to acute stressors immediately, remove you from danger, and then calm down again—although as we'll see, especially if the acute stressor is severe enough, that doesn't always happen.

Chronic stress is long-term or repeated over time. A demanding job with a boss who keeps you late every day is a chronic stressor. Caring for a family member with dementia is a chronic stressor. Living in a high-crime area or in poverty, or being stuck in an unstable or abusive home environment, are chronic stressors. Chronic stress is a very common cause of inflammation.

WHEN THE STRESS NEVER STOPS

A *persistent stressor* is any condition that creates a hostile environment for your body over a long period of time.

Some of the stressors I've mentioned, like job stress or caring for a loved one with a major illness, are persistent stressors. These aren't one-time events that cause your fight-or-flight response to turn on all at once, then turn off again. Instead, they create constantly stressful conditions you can't escape from.

Remember the broken thermostat? A persistent stressor is like an open window. Cold air constantly blows over the thermostat's sensor, making it think the room is much colder than it really is. So the thermostat never shuts off. It keeps the heat running all the time. There's no single moment when the heating system breaks down, but over time, the situation gets worse and worse.

The same snowball effect can happen in your body.

Persistent stressors are usually less obvious than traumatic events. You can rarely look back on a single moment and say, "That's when it all started!" Your body just never gets a break—like a new parent who never gets a full night's sleep after having a child.

When stress is constant, or when it's repeated or you can't get away from it, your body never has a chance to recover. The stress response stays turned on. Systems get more and more out of balance. That's one reason that stress experienced early in life (sometimes before you're even born!) can spiral into serious mental health symptoms later on—and why early-life stress often has a more damaging effect on your system than stress experienced as an adult.[25]

Perhaps the most disruptive, and paradoxical, effect of chronic stress is that it can damage your stress "off" switch. Normally, when you experience a stressor, your body responds, then resets. Chronic stress can make your body less and less able to turn the stress response off.

Result? More and more build-up of stress hormones like cortisol in the body, leading to long-term damage and inflammation.[26]

Persistent stressors can cause symptoms and effects that show up much later in your life, so much later that it can be hard to remember where or when the symptoms started. Fortunately, it's possible to treat the damage itself—including the inflammation. Even symptoms that have been part of your life for years can be improved.

WHEN EVERYTHING CHANGES IN A MOMENT

Unlike a persistent stressor, a traumatic event is a single incident so stressful it pushes your fight-or-flight response into high gear instantaneously.

---

25 Sonia J. Lupien et al., "Effects of Stress throughout the Lifespan on the Brain, Behaviour and Cognition," *Nature Reviews Neuroscience* 10 (April 29, 2009): 434–45, https://doi.org/10.1038/nrn2639.

26 Sheldon Cohen et al., "Chronic Stress, Glucocorticoid Receptor Resistance, Inflammation, and Disease Risk," *Proceedings of the National Academy of Sciences USA* 109, no. 16 (April 2, 2012): 5995–99, https://doi.org/10.1073/pnas.1118355109.

Also unlike persistent stressors, you generally know right away when you've experienced a traumatic event. Traumatic events often involve physical injury to yourself or others, including having major surgery or witnessing someone's death. A traumatic event makes you feel powerful emotions, like fear or horror about what's happening.

Car accidents are traumatic events. Being assaulted or seeing someone else hurt, losing a loved one, and being hospitalized can all be traumatic events. Being forced out of your home as a refugee is another.

And keep in mind: many, many people live through traumatic events, even though they may not label them that way. While a war or a major injury are obviously traumatic, many events that seem "normal" can be traumatic as well. If you are yelled at by your boss in front of your coworkers, that is traumatic. Being pushed around by a bully at school is traumatic.

Whether something is traumatic isn't about how severe it *seems*. All of these are traumatic events because they are single incidents that can ratchet your stress response up to "full blast" all at once. Whether a particular event has that effect on a particular person depends on their unique stress resilience—their ability to "bounce back"—which is the result of their genetics and their environment.

In the thermostat analogy, a traumatic event is like a mouse chewing through the wiring. The damage doesn't happen over a long period of time. It's immediate. The system goes wrong the moment the wire is severed.

What we're learning about traumatic events is that they're not always over when they're over. In some cases, the body recovers the way it's supposed to, and everything goes back to balance—but in other cases, the stress response is so hyped up that it doesn't know to shut back down.

You're probably familiar with PTSD. PTSD, or post-traumatic stress disorder, occurs when someone continues to reexperience a traumatic event over and over in their mind, or experience traumatic emotions and feelings long after the event. Even though the traumatic experience is over, the mind and body can't let it go. The stress response stays in the "on" position.

Even though the mouse isn't there chewing on the wire anymore, the system doesn't come back online. Until the wire is reconnected, the furnace can't work properly.

Even traumatic events that occurred decades ago can still be causing damage. Think about Camilla. The trauma she experienced as a refugee happened so long ago that she can barely remember it. But the effects are still present in her body and brain. If anything, they are getting worse.

GENETICS AND SELF-COMPASSION

Interestingly, not everyone who experiences a traumatic event—not even everyone who experiences *the same* traumatic event—will develop PTSD or develop it to the same extent. Similarly, not everyone who experiences fear develops an anxiety disorder. The reasons range from genetic differences to support systems and childhood experiences, but scientists have recently discovered another reason. It's called *neuropeptide Y* (NPY).

I'm not going to get into all the scientific details here, but suffice it to say: NPY makes your brain more resilient against stress, and some people naturally produce more of it than others.[27] Think of it as another reason not to blame yourself or feel ashamed of your symptoms. It's possible your brain just makes less of this compound than some other people's.

27 Zhifeng Zhou et al., "Genetic Variation in Human *NPY* Expression Affects Stress Response and Emotion," *Nature* 452 (April 2008): 997–1001, https://doi.org/10.1038/nature06858.

STRESS AND INFLAMMATION

Whether it's caused by a single traumatic event or persistent stressors, once the stress response is turned on, inflammation is the result. Over time, if the inflammation keeps building, it can lead to problems that seem less and less related to the original cause.

Like I said before, you don't have to remember all the details of the biology. What's important is that inflammation causes different kinds of damage in your body as time goes on. These different kinds of damage can lead to very different symptoms.

LOCALIZED DAMAGE

Localized damage is the first stage of inflammation. *Localized* just means that the damage is in one specific location and hasn't spread.

When we talked about cutting your finger, that was localized inflammation. It occurred in one specific place on your body: your finger. Because that was a minor injury, the inflammation did its job and then went away.

But remember how we said that the immune system is like knights guarding your castle? Knights are great when they are fighting, but they can leave one heck of a mess when the battle is over.

Imagine your castle humming along on a normal day. Everyone inside the castle is doing their jobs. The bakers are baking. The blacksmith is making swords and armor. A farmer drives a cart full of vegetables back toward the kitchens. Life is going well.

Suddenly, a trumpet blares! Invaders are attacking the north wall! From deep inside the castle, soldiers come running to the defense.

A week-long battle ensues, but finally...success! The invaders are turned back. The soldiers take off their armor and head back to their quarters to rest.

But as the castle tries to get back to normal activity, you discover that everything is not the same as it was before. The place where the knights were fighting is now a wasteland. They left trash everywhere. The ground has been pounded into slushy mud. The castle walls have been burnt and broken, even on the inside. An entire section of the castle is going to have to be rebuilt and repaired. Someone's going to have to clean up all the waste before it turns into toxic goop and infects the crops.

A battle that rages in one place for a long time leaves behind trash and destruction. Immune cells are no different. They fight for you, but they also create waste and damage. Specifically, immune cells leave behind something called *reactive oxygen species*. You might have also heard them referred to as *free radicals*.

It's surprising to think that any kind of oxygen could cause harm. After all, you can only survive a few minutes without it. Your cells need oxygen, too, or they'll die.

But oxygen is also one of the most destructive chemicals on the planet.

When immune cells fight off invaders, they spew out oxygen compounds called "free radicals" as waste. These compounds are called "reactive" because they react easily with other molecules, breaking them down. When free-floating oxygen compounds get out into your bloodstream, they can damage DNA and break down proteins your body needs to live. This is sometimes called *oxidative stress*.

These free radicals can also destroy cells. When those cells are invaders, that's mostly a good thing—but it's not so great when the process turns against healthy cells that you need.

If you've ever heard of antioxidants, that's actually related to this free radical effect. The word antioxidant literally means "against oxygen" or "something that inhibits oxygen." Foods like blueberries and dark, leafy greens are good for you in part because they block the reactivity of the free-floating, destructive oxygen molecules.

Unfortunately, once the inflammation cycle speeds up, a cup of blueberries and a spinach salad aren't enough on their own. (They do still help though.) If the stressor is extreme enough or continues long enough, the problem starts to spread through your whole system. Then the damage is no longer localized.

SYSTEMIC INFLAMMATION

When inflammation becomes *systemic*, that means it's started to occur throughout the body. It's no longer localized.

Remember how I said that the stress response was complex—that it requires several different systems working together? The downside to this complexity is that breakdowns in the system can also come from lots of different directions.

Stress can directly affect the immune system, reducing the number of killer cells—the immune cells that fight off invaders.[28] That in turn makes you more susceptible to infection, which causes more stress.

But stress can also cause inflammation more indirectly. For one thing, being stressed is exhausting. It tends to redirect energy and resources toward the systems that are responding to the stress, leaving you with less energy for everything else—including fighting infection and keeping yourself healthy. And as you already know, stress increases hormones like cortisol, which can actively damage cells if it circulates in the blood for too long.[29]

However it happens, when inflammation becomes systemic, it causes damage far and wide, and you find yourself with symptoms that may seem like they've got nothing to do with stress at all. Rheumatoid arthritis, multiple sclerosis, lupus, heart disease, asthma...the list is too long to repeat here.

And once inflammation is systemic, it requires a systemic approach to treatment as well.

---

28 C. J. Chan, M. J. Smyth, and L. Martinet, "Molecular Mechanisms of Natural Killer Cell Activation in Response to Cellular Stress," *Cell Death & Differentiation* 21 (January 2014): 5–14, https://doi.org/10.1038/cdd.2013.26.

29 Kirstin Aschbacher et al., "Good Stress, Bad Stress, and Oxidative Stress: Insights from Anticipatory Cortisol Reactivity," *Psychoneuroendocrinology* 38, no. 9 (September 2013): 1698–1708, https://doi.org/10.1016/j.psyneuen.2013.02.004.

Infection Not Required

Do you remember that scary movie with the tagline, "The call is coming from *inside the house*"? That can happen with the stress cycle too. You don't have to be exposed to any infection or external cause of inflammation: the trigger that starts the inflammatory cycle can come from within.

This is what's been called the *sterile immune response*. Sterile doesn't mean it's clean like an operating room. Sterile means you haven't been infected from outside.

What happens instead is that your body starts to see *your own cells* as intruders.

This can happen for a number of reasons, but chronic stress is a big one. When you experience chronic stress, your cells get stressed too.

Have you ever been so stressed that someone told you, "Wow, you look tired," or even, "You are not yourself today"? That's what happens with your cells. They don't "look like" themselves to your immune system. As a result, your immune system treats them as intruders. It sends the alert: we've been invaded! And the inflammatory response kicks on.

When your immune system identifies a cell as an invader, it gets a "mug shot" of that cell to show all the other immune responders, so they can ID the invader too. When it's your own cell, that's bad news. Now your immune system thinks that at least some of your own cells are bad guys.

As the immune system goes around trying to fight off this invasion, it sees more and more of these "bad guys" (because they're your own cells), and kicks its response up a notch. And finds more cells. And kicks up a notch.

Just to top it all off, with your immune system busy fighting your own cells, it has fewer resources to fight real invaders, making you more likely to get an infection. (That's why you often get sick when you're stressed out or really busy.)

This is part of why it's so important to disrupt the stress cycle as well as fight the inflammation directly.

LEAKY BRAIN

The third way that inflammation causes damage in the body is called *leaky brain.*

I know, it sounds terrifying.

I honestly don't even like talking about it. But it's critical to understanding how inflammation impacts mental health.

In Chapter Two, we talked about the blood-brain barrier and how it's really more of a filter. The blood-brain barrier keeps bad guys out of the brain and neurotransmitters in. In general, it keeps the brain and body separate. Even if you get medicine delivered directly into your vein through an IV, there's still a good chance it won't reach your brain.

Because of the barrier, the brain has its own homeostasis and its own immune system. It's like your brain is on lockdown, 24 hours a day. Access is tightly controlled.

Leaky brain happens when inflammation pokes holes in the blood-brain barrier. The tightly controlled access is compromised. More of the body's blood and cells and molecules get into the brain. Suddenly, the brain and the body are interacting in an unfiltered way.

Some of the cells that get through are immune cells, like white blood cells. Where white blood cells go, inflammation follows. As inflammation in the body increases, so does inflammation in the brain.

The brain then responds by increasing its own immune response. Normally, that would be contained by the blood-brain barrier. But because of the holes in the barrier, the inflammation leaks back into the body and triggers more inflammation there. Once the barrier starts to break down, inflammation in the brain and body set each other off. The leaks increase, and the barrier becomes weaker. It's a vicious cycle.

HELP ON THE WAY

Systemic inflammation, imbalances in the HPA axis, and leaky brain often occur together. Traumatic events and persistent stressors lead to chronic inflammation, and symptoms start piling on top of one another.

Put it all together, and the process can sound scary and depressing. After all, who wants a "leaky" brain?

It's important to understand the basic science behind stress and inflammation because understanding the real problem is the first step to finding real solutions. If you're suffering from mental health problems and haven't been able to find any answers, chronic inflammation may be to blame.

Rest assured: there are solutions, and they are within your grasp.

RESETTING THE TEMPERATURE

If chronic inflammation is an out-of-control thermostat, Camilla's has been set on high for decades.

When she was woken in the middle of the night as a child and forced to leave her home, she experienced a traumatic event. Her months as a refugee, followed by years of poverty, acted as persistent stressors. And her PTSD was the "stressor within," pushing her system into overdrive again and again.

Her stress response originally helped her get through difficult, terrifying events. But it never turned off, and the chronic inflammation cycle was set in motion.

Unfortunately, her body couldn't send her a text message. It couldn't say, "Hey, I've got chronic inflammation here!" The body speaks to us through symptoms. Camilla's body spoke to her through pain, trouble sleeping, and deep, punishing fatigue.

Once she realized that chronic inflammation was an underlying factor beneath all of her seemingly disconnected symptoms, she had a lot more options and could make better choices. She started to look for therapies that would help reset her system. She realized that she needed to slow down the chronic inflammation cycle enough to let her body finally heal. After literally decades of increasing pain and suffering, Camilla finally had hope.

We'll see Camilla again, later in her healing journey, as she discovers approaches that treat her real problem, not just her symptoms. Treating her underlying inflammation has given her new options and an improved quality of life. Knowing what was really going on was her first step toward gaining control over her symptoms.

AND NOW: THE MOMENT WE'VE ALL BEEN WAITING FOR

Okay, take a second to pause.

Breathe.

Let it out.

And give yourself a break.

You won't remember all the science from these chapters. That's okay.

You will probably have to come back and be like, "What was that HPA thing again?" All good.

In the end, that doesn't matter because while understanding is great, it's not the point.

Getting better—*feeling* better and *living* better: that's the point.

And that, my friends, is where we are headed.

Like Camilla, we all need the best possible tools to support our bodies and brains in regulating and healing the inflammatory cycle. Modern life is hard. It's complex and complicated, and it's all too easy for us to get stuck with chronic stress and inflammation, even if we never experienced childhood trauma or severe traumatic events.

It's not enough to just manage your symptoms. Reducing the day-to-day impact of your symptoms can be life-changing, but it doesn't fix the underlying problem. You need ways to slow down or stop the inflammation so the body can heal itself.

From here on out, that's what this book is about: tools and solutions. Actionable approaches that you can use to achieve your highest-possible quality of life.

And believe me, that means *you*. You can feel better. You can choose tools and solutions that work for your life and your symptoms. You can take back your life. Feeling and living better isn't just for other people. It's for you.

Maybe not every single approach in this book is for you. Feel free to pick and choose. Maybe you start in one place and end up somewhere else. Great! This is the part where you get to take control and get your health back, for yourself.

So—what are we waiting for?

TL;DR

→ Your body maintains its balance and health through a process called *homeostasis*, which keeps the body's systems within acceptable ranges.

→ Chronic inflammation is like a broken thermostat. Instead of turning off once the stress, illness, or injury is over, it stays on. That wreaks all kinds of havoc in the body and brain.

→ Two kinds of stress contribute to inflammation: chronic or persistent (long-term) stress and acute (one-time) stress. Traumatic events are acute stressors. Ongoing work or family issues are persistent stressors.

→ Inflammation can cause *local* damage to cells and tissues in one area of the body. Over time, it can create *systemic* issues throughout the body. That's one reason that inflammation can show up in a lot of different ways.

→ Systems in the body called the SAM system and the HPA axis are the body's short-term (SAM) and long-term (HPA) stress responders. Chronic stressors and traumatic events can affect their healthy functioning, and these systems can throw the body out of balance.

TAKING ACTION AGAINST INFLAMMATION

We're going to jump right into the inflammation-fighting approaches in the next chapter, but first, I want to tell you a story.

I recently went to visit an old friend in Northern California. I was really looking forward to the trip, and I knew she was looking forward to us spending some quality time together as well. So I was surprised when I drove up to her house. Two big vans were parked haphazardly across her driveway, and her front lawn was littered with ladders and coiled lengths of hose.

As soon as I got out of the car, I heard voices and looked up to see where they were coming from. Half a dozen guys in bright yellow shirts were milling around on top of her flat roof, wiping away sweat and laying down big strips of green sod.

It looked like they were...*gardening* her roof, although that didn't make sense.

At that moment, I saw my friend waving at me from the edge of the roof. "Hi hi hi! Up here!" she called. I left my bags in the car, carefully climbed one of the ladders leaning against the house, and popped up into a chaotic scene, two guys right in front of me yelling at each other about getting the edges lined up and another two struggling to pull another strip of sod up a ladder. They *were* gardening her roof.

After hugs and a bit of small talk, she gestured around and asked, "What do you think?"

"It's nice," I started, then paused. "But...why?"

She laughed. "Yeah, it looks a bit odd, but it's fire prevention."

Suddenly it made sense. Her neighborhood had barely escaped the wildfires the previous year, so now she was going to do whatever she could to protect her house.

"Is that the reason for the rocks too?" I nodded toward the twelve-foot ring of gravel surrounding her house where bushes used to be.

"Yep. It's a fire break. You surround the house with stuff that's not flammable. If there's nothing for the fire to consume, it's less likely to get close, and the house will be safe. I'm putting green stuff on the roof because it doesn't catch easily, and I set up a sprinkler right next to the house to spray down the walls if necessary. I'm as prepared as I can be."

PREVENT, CONTAIN, RECOVER

Watching my friend prepare her house for wildfires made me think about inflammation and how we manage it. In fact, the approaches and techniques I'm going to teach you in this book look a lot like fire management strategies.

Wildfire management isn't just about dumping water on active fires. It's about protecting our homes and neighborhoods as best we can, containing and mitigating a fire once it's broken out, and then recovering as individuals and as a community after the fire is over.

That's even what firefighters call it: recovery. And that's what this book is about too.

Living in the modern world is like living in wildfire country. Everything in our lives, from our jobs to our childhood experiences to the noise in our environment, has the potential to cause stress and inflammation. And like people who live near wildfire danger, our best approach is to protect ourselves as well as we can, mitigate and control the damage once inflammation is occurring, and work toward full recovery with all the tools in our toolbox.

The good news is that no matter how long you've lived with chronic inflammation, no matter how severe your symptoms, no matter how hard it's been, you can take meaningful action to improve your life. The rest of this book will introduce you to the evidence-based tools to start you in the right direction.

FROM EVERYDAY HABITS TO CUTTING-EDGE TECHNOLOGIES

Every recovery approach, tool, or method I discuss in this book has the potential to meaningfully impact your life. Some take substantial time and commitment, while others can have an effect almost immediately. Some you can do in your sweatpants in the living room, while others require help from a licensed therapist or your doctor.

Some involve everyday lifestyle changes. Others involve innovative new technologies.

Section Two will introduce you to protection and prevention strategies that can help mitigate, or contain, the damage caused by inflammation. Section Three will describe mental health practices that can also contain, reduce, or control inflammation and its symptoms. And Section Four (the most exciting section, in my opinion) will introduce you to cutting-edge recovery technologies.

The treatments and technologies I address later in the book might seem more innovative and faster acting. And that's true. In some ways, the everyday habits I address in Section Two are steps on a long journey, whereas the "accelerated" approaches I talk about later on are like jumping on a bullet train to your destination.

It can be tempting to just jump into the high-tech, fast-moving solutions right away. And if that works for you, and you have access to those interventions, do it!

However, even the most high-tech, innovative, cutting-edge technologies and therapies have the best chance of working if they are built on a solid, secure foundation. That's why I'll start with the everyday changes you can start making today.

In the end, the measure of how successful a fire response was is not just whether the fire is put out. The real test is whether the people in the community can get their lives back. In other words, it's not just about managing. It's about thriving.

And that's what I want for you too.

REPAIRING YOUR ECOSYSTEM

The Inflammation-Fighting Power of Everyday Practices

One reason wildfires rage out of control is that dry brush builds up in the understory. Dead saplings, fallen leaves, and dried-out branches catch fire far more easily than living trees. A forest that's full of those things will catch like tinder and spread extremely quickly.

Putting out a wildfire in that situation takes longer. There's more damage and destruction. The fire burns hotter and is harder to contain.

Managing depression, anxiety, and other mental health challenges while eating poorly, living a sedentary lifestyle, or never getting enough sleep is like trying to fight a wildfire in a forest full of dried tinder.

The bad news is that many of us are living this way. The good news is that even small, simple, everyday changes can start to "clear the brush," leaving your forest healthier and calming inflammation so you have a chance to get better.

In fact, these practices go way beyond just clearing the brush. They help you turn your body from a tinder box to a thriving ecosystem.

A thriving forest ecosystem is fire resistant and, maybe more importantly, it's set up to *withstand* and *survive* a fire. Fire is natural. A healthy forest will bounce back from a wildfire healthier than ever.

A forest that is struggling for basic resources burns harder, but it also doesn't recover as quickly. It will be more exposed to the next fire—and it's more likely that there will be another fire. With each episode of damage, the forest becomes less and less able to recover before the next one.

STRUGGLING FOR RESOURCES

Our bodies work the same way. We need basic, fundamental resources in order to survive and thrive. We need nutrients to feed our cells, movement to keep our blood supplying every nook and cranny of our bodies, and sleep to reset our minds and repair our organs.

These basic resources make up the foundation of our mental and physical health. Without them, we cannot repair the damage caused by stress and inflammation. We become like the depleted forest: more susceptible to damage and less able to recover. We fall into a cycle of decreasing function of our cells, organs, minds, bodies, and, eventually, our quality of life.

Many of us are living in debt when it comes to our basic resources. Think about the last time you didn't move much for a whole week or the last time you ate too much junk food. The way you felt afterward was your body struggling for resources.

When you add stress and inflammation, the problem gets worse. Your body uses extra resources to rebuild and repair itself when it's sick or damaged. People suffering from mental or physical health problems need even more basic resources than others.

Short version? If you want to give your body and brain the best possible chance at getting healthier, you need to start by giving it the resources to repair itself.

The most important resources for your recovery are good nutrition, exercise, and sleep. Or, as I like to call them, fuel, movement, and rest. Together, improvements in these three areas of your life will create a thriving body ecosystem, a stable baseline from which to heal.

Fuel powers your cells and gives your body the energy it needs to function and repair itself. Some kinds of food are fuels that actively reduce inflammation in the body, while others can actually worsen it.

Movement increases blood flow, allowing the fuel to reach your cells. It also clears out waste and increases levels of anti-inflammatory chemicals in your body and brain.

Rest allows your body and brain the time and energy needed to repair themselves. Lack of rest increases inflammation, but getting enough rest pushes you back into balance.

The best part about fuel, movement, and rest is that they are things you can do yourself. No appointments or equipment needed. You can take charge of your own mental health and reduce inflammation right now. Today.

And you don't have to run a marathon or become a vegan chef to do it.

THRIVE BIG WITH SMALL WINS

It can be hard to talk about some of these topics, especially the "d" word and the "e" word (diet and exercise), because there is just so much noise out there. Everybody from athletes and actors to your next-door neighbor is trying to tell you what to eat or which new exercise is the "magic bullet."

I've heard it all myself. The nagging. The pressure. Especially when you're not feeling well—then everyone seems to have advice for you.

Suddenly everybody and their sister has ideas about how much you should be exercising and how you'd feel so much better if you would just come to their "boot camp" class, or their spin class, or whatever else they swear by.

That is not what I'm offering here. This section of the book isn't about fads or extreme diets. It's about making realistic, achievable, *evidence-supported* everyday adjustments that directly address chronic inflammation and add up to major improvements in mental health.

In fact, let's pause for a moment before we start talking about solutions.

I'd like you to close your eyes, take a deep breath, and clear your mind of everything you've ever heard about diets, exercise, and sleep. Just forget all of it.

Instead of all that, I'm going to give you what I like to call the *min/max*: the minimum effort to get the greatest benefit. You will learn the smallest things you can do to get the biggest real outcomes in terms of stress, inflammation, and mental health.

By the end of this section, you will have a whole toolbox full of evidence-supported "small wins" to decrease chronic inflammation and improve your own mental health.

It only takes small changes to add up to big impacts. You can do these things in the privacy of your living room or out with friends. You can stack one small win on top of another until you've achieved big, lasting mental health gains. Before you know it, your ecosystem will be thriving again.

Most importantly, everything in this section, like everything in this book, is supported by science and proven to directly impact chronic inflammation. No fads allowed.

Let's start with fuel.

CHAPTER FOUR

FUEL FOR BRAIN HEALTH

Stephanie has started parking down the block from her daughter's school and waiting for her there. She doesn't like to pull up to the front door these days because she doesn't want the other moms to see her shaking.

It's been five years since her accident, but she still can't get over the panic that rises in her gut every time she hears a loud horn or sees someone run a red light. Every time she makes a left turn, she finds herself breathing hard and almost unable to stay on the road.

Everyone tells her she should be "over it" by now. She's physically fine. She knows that. But it's not that simple. Every time she seems to have it under control, she sees a black truck or has to decide whether to go through a yellow light, and then she's thrown right back into the panic again.

At least that's understandable though. Feeling dread when she's driving makes sense. What doesn't make sense to her is what has been happening in her stomach recently.

When the symptoms first started, they were unpredictable. She'd get cramps after eating sometimes, or she'd be hit by a sudden need to run to the bathroom, often at the worst possible times. Like out on the field, coaching her kids' ultimate games. One time, she barely made it, and ever since then, she gets nervous when she's too far away from a restroom. It's humiliating, even if no one else knows.

And it's not getting better. If anything, over the past six months, it's gotten worse and worse. Now her cramps are sometimes so painful they disrupt her entire day. She has to lie on the couch with a heating pad, fatigued and sweating, hoping the feeling passes before she has to be somewhere.

She's started looking at food differently. Even though she's hungry, she doesn't know what foods she can trust. Her energy level is lower than it's ever been. She can't eat anything without worrying about what the consequences might be. Some days, the pain in her gut is so bad she can't stand up straight. Often, it comes with headaches and nausea.

Before all this started, she didn't realize how important it was to be able to eat without thinking about it. Being stuck in this loop of not knowing what she can eat, forcing herself to get enough food, and then suffering has made her hard to live with. She's impatient with her kids and partner. She feels irritable most of the time. She struggles to keep up with the busy pace of her life.

She finally goes to her doctor, and he tells her she's developed celiac disease. Apparently, whenever she eats gluten (a protein that's in wheat and some other grains), it's actually damaging her intestines. It's an immune reaction rooted in inflammation.

What the doctor is saying seems so unfair to her—she can't even eat bread! As if the stress and anxiety from the accident weren't bad enough by itself. She was planning to get back into the art community after the kids graduate. She and her husband were finally going to travel. But how can she travel when she never knows what her stomach will be doing tomorrow?

Her world used to revolve around her family and her work. Now it revolves around the monster in her gut. Until it's gone, or at least under some kind of control, Stephanie knows she won't be able to get back to her old self.

NOT ALL FUEL IS CREATED EQUAL

When your body is feeling healthy and well, it's easy to not pay attention to what you're eating. Maybe you grab a snack as you walk out the door or pick up some takeout on the way home. But as Stephanie learned, life gets a lot more complicated when you have to think about every single thing you put in your mouth.

What Stephanie is learning is that not all foods—not all fuels—are created equal. And that's especially true if you're suffering from inflammation-related issues.

It's a lot like what happens with cars. I honestly don't know a lot about cars, but I have a friend who's a car guy. He always has two or three "projects" parked in his driveway or his garage, and he loves to work on cars and talk about cars, so I end up hearing a lot about them.

One of his favorite cars is an ancient diesel pickup truck he bought in college. It's huge and loud, but according to him, more powerful than a modern F-150. I'm going to take his word on that one.

A while ago, I read an article about people putting used cooking oil in diesel engines as fuel. I showed him the article and asked if he'd heard of that.

I thought he'd be impressed that I was learning about cars on my own, but he wasn't. He actually rolled his eyes at me. "Look," he said, "sure, you can run your diesel engine on used cooking oil. But have you seen the stuff you clean off your frying pan? That oil is full of *gunk*."

It turns out if you put used cooking oil in your diesel engine, it will run. For a while. Maybe even for a long time. But not forever. My friend learned that the hard way, back in college. He and his friends decided to drive across the country in his truck, and since they were broke college kids, they decided to save money by collecting used cooking oil and filling the truck with that. They started out full of excitement, with a truck bed full of gallon jugs of oil.

They ended up stranded in the middle of the desert.

Why? Because over time, the "gunk," as my friend called it, built up in the engine and brought the whole thing to a shuddering stop. What surprised me most when he told me the story was that clean cooking oil ends up being almost as bad. It doesn't have bits and pieces in it, but it's just not the fuel the engine was meant to run on.

Like a diesel engine, your body can run for a surprising amount of time on bad fuel. But if you put fast food and Twinkies in your body for years, it's like putting cooking oil in your diesel truck. Over time, you're going to break down.

In order to repair your body and brain, you need better fuel sources: foods high in beneficial nutrients. What your body runs best on. And not just your body, but your brain as well. Most people know that eating well is important for body health. What's less well known is that it's just as important for brain health—and thus mental health.

GUT FEELINGS

"I've got a gut feeling about this."

"What does your gut tell you?"

"Trust your gut."

It's no accident that we use the word "gut" when we talk about our feelings and our decisions. It's the same reason your stomach ties in knots when you're about to give a presentation, and you often feel a sense of "something wrong" in your stomach when you're faced with a choice you don't like.

That's your gut-brain axis in action.

Your gut has its own nervous system, often called the *second brain*, which can operate independently from the brain in your head. This second brain in your gut is known as the *enteric nervous system* ("enteric" means anything to do with the intestines). It's incredibly weird to think of your intestines as a thinking organ, but that's what the science is showing us.

The second brain in your gut contains millions of neurons and is in constant communication with your brain—the main one inside your skull.[30] This communication happens through chemicals and electrical signals, and it can affect your mood, your emotions, and even your decision-making processes.[31]

So when people say, "trust your gut," there's a reason.

And the communication goes both ways. Why does that matter? Because it means gut health can directly impact brain health, including brain inflammation.

One study even found that problems with gut health led to disruption of neurotransmitters in the brain and, from there, to eventual cognitive decline. In other words, poor gut health can lead to Alzheimer's.[32]

How does this connection work?

The first thing to understand about the gut is that it's absolutely chock-full of bacteria. When I say chock-full, I mean it's *mostly* bacteria. In fact, you and I are mostly made up of bacteria.

Single-celled organisms (mostly bacteria) outnumber your own cells in your body ten to one.

Ten to one.

To put it another way, your body is 90 percent single-celled organisms, and only 10 percent, well, *you*.

Most of these bacteria live in your gut, and they make up what's called your *microbiota*. That basically means "the part of you that's made up of microscoping things."

The absolute strangest thing about these, well, *strangers* living in your body is that they are necessary to your well-being. Unlike the kind of bacteria or other single-celled organisms that cause dis-

30   Marilia Carabotti et al., "The Gut-Brain Axis: Interactions between Enteric Microbiota, Central and Enteric Nervous Systems," *Annals of Gastroenterology* 28, no. 2 (April–June 2015): 203–209, https://www.ncbi.nlm.nih.gov/pmc/articles/PMC4367209/.

31   Jeremy Appleton, "The Gut-Brain Axis: Influence of Microbiota on Mood and Mental Health," *Integrative Medicine* 17, no. 4 (August 2018): 28–32, https://www.ncbi.nlm.nih.gov/pmc/articles/PMC6469458/.

32   Diane Bairamian et al., "Microbiota in Neuroinflammation and Synaptic Dysfunction: A Focus on Alzheimer's Disease," *Molecular Neurodegeneration* 17 (March 2022): 19, https://doi.org/10.1186/s13024-022-00522-2.

ease, these ones help your body stay healthy—mentally as well as physically.

In one study, for example, researchers found that people with depression had much lower overall levels of gut bacteria than people without depression.[33]

But the evidence for this connection goes way beyond one study. One of the largest-scale reviews of human studies ever conducted found a clear connection between microbiota and psychiatric disorders of all kinds. Study after study showed that people with mental health challenges had notable differences in their gut compared to control-group participants.[34]

What you eat can powerfully influence the health of your gut and the diversity and well-being of your microbiota. And as if that weren't enough, food choices can directly affect inflammation as well.

THE INFLAMMATION CONNECTION

What you eat has a direct impact on inflammation in your body and brain, and that impact can go either way. Your food can be a powerful anti-inflammatory ally...or another driver in the pro-inflammatory cycle.

Researchers have found that typical Western food choices heat up inflammation in the body.[35] That means that a lot of us are starting out at a high-inflammation baseline.

On the other side, anti-inflammatory foods reduce inflammation. One study found, for example, that fruit and vegetable intake was

---

33 Akash Kumar et al., "Gut Microbiota in Anxiety and Depression: Unveiling the Relationships and Management Options," *Pharmaceuticals* 16, no. 4 (April 9, 2023): 565, https://doi.org/10.3390/ph16040565.

34 Carmen Grau-Del Valle et al., "Association between Gut Microbiota and Psychiatric Disorders: A Systematic Review," *Frontiers in Psychology* 14 (August 2, 2023), https://doi.org/10.3389/fpsyg.2023.1215674.

35 Dario Giugliano, Antonio Ceriello, and Katherine Esposito, "The Effects of Diet on Inflammation: Emphasis on the Metabolic Syndrome," *Journal of the American College of Cardiology* 48, no. 4 (August 15, 2006): 677–85, https://doi.org/10.1016/j.jacc.2006.03.052.

directly related to the levels of C-reactive protein in the blood.[36] C-reactive protein is a key marker of inflammation in the body that doctors use to predict heart attack risk and other conditions linked to inflammation. Eating enough fruit and vegetables reduces it.

Beyond just baseline inflammation, though, our food choices can also have a profound effect on inflammation-related diseases. Anti-inflammatory foods have been shown to reduce and slow the development of Parkinson's symptoms, and brand-new research has found that a pro-inflammatory diet creates an increased risk of relapse for people with multiple sclerosis.[37]

THE PLASTICS PROBLEM

Just to complicate things, it turns out that it's not just what we eat that's important. What we eat it *with*, or *from*, can matter just as much.

Case in point: plastic.

Plastics are everywhere. They get in our food (from Tupperware, cooking utensils, and flatware), in our water (from unfiltered water sources, water bottles, plastic water filters), and on *and even in* our bodies (from polyester clothing, bedding, shampoos, and other sources).[38]

Many plastics are made up of chemicals that are extremely harmful to the body over time. This is so much the case that some

---

36 Xiang Gao, Odilia I. Bermudez, and Katherine L. Tucker, "Plasma C-Reactive Protein and Homocysteine Concentrations Are Related to Frequent Fruit and Vegetable Intake in Hispanic and Non-Hispanic White Elders," *Journal of Nutrition* 134, no. 4 (April 2004): 913–18, https://doi.org/10.1093/jn/134.4.913.

37 Stefania Kalampokini et al., "Nonpharmacological Modulation of Chronic Inflammation in Parkinson's Disease: Role of Diet Interventions," *Parkinson's Disease* 2019 (August 25, 2019): 7535472, https://doi.org/10.1155%2F2019%2F7535472; and Alice M. Saul et al., "A Pro-Inflammatory Diet in People with Multiple Sclerosis Is Associated with an Increased Rate of Relapse and Increased FLAIR Lesion Volume on MRI in Early Multiple Sclerosis: A Prospective Cohort Study," *Multiple Sclerosis Journal* 29, no. 8 (July 2023): 1012–23, https://doi.org/10.1177/13524585231167739.

38 UN Environment Programme, *Chemicals in Plastics: A Technical Report* (Geneva: United Nations Environment Programme, 2023), https://www.unep.org/resources/report/chemicals-plastics-technical-report.

countries—including the United Kingdom, Canada, and the European Union—have passed laws to make plastic production illegal.[39]

One of the biggest offenders is water bottles. The World Health Organization just launched a worldwide investigation on bottled water after a test revealed that *nine out of ten bottles of water contain plastic contamination.*[40]

So am I saying that drinking from a plastic water bottle can be harmful? Unfortunately, yes.

A water bottle looks solid, but if you zoomed in with a microscope, you'd see tons of tiny, loose pieces of plastic, called *microplastics*, that come off the bottle like sawdust off a project in woodshop.

That microplastic "dust" gets into your body and interrupts healthy cell functions.[41] Some microplastics can look like hormones, like estrogen and testosterone, so they send the wrong signals and disrupt normal body functions. Certain plastics, such as BPA and phthalates, have been linked to everything from breast cancer and birth defects to obesity and heart disease.[42]

What can you do? Limit your plastic use wherever you can, especially near your food.

The same food choices impact mental health symptoms as well. Dietary inflammatory index, a measure of how inflammation-causing your food is, has been associated with higher risk of depression and anxiety, and lower well-being, in adults.[43]

In other words, food can improve your health, but it can also be

---

39   Annie Greenberg, "Plastic Free July: How 20 Countries Are Taking Action," Sustainable Ocean Alliance, July 5, 2022, https://www.soalliance.org/soablog/plastic-free-july-20-countries-taking-action.

40   Sherri A. Mason, Victoria G. Welch, and Joseph Neratko, "Synthetic Polymer Contamination in Bottled Water," *Frontiers in Chemistry* 6 (September 11, 2018), https://doi.org/10.3389/fchem.2018.00407.

41   Claudia Campanale et al., "A Detailed Review Study on Potential Effects of Microplastics and Additives of Concern on Human Health," *International Journal of Environmental Research and Public Health* 17, no. 4 (February 13, 2020): 1212, https://doi.org/10.3390/ijerph17041212.

42   Anna H. Wu et al., "Urinary Phthalate Exposures and Risk of Breast Cancer: The Multiethnic Cohort Study," *Breast Cancer Research* 23 (2021): 44, https://doi.org/10.1186/s13058-021-01419-6.

43   Catherine M. Phillips et al., "Dietary Inflammatory Index and Mental Health: A Cross-Sectional Analysis of the Relationship with Depressive Symptoms, Anxiety and Well-Being in Adults," *Clinical Nutrition* 37, no. 5 (October 2018): 1485–91, https://doi.org/10.1016/j.clnu.2017.08.029.

another stressor that contributes to inflammatory damage. Some foods help your body repair itself, while others damage cells, activate the immune response, or even directly create inflammation. Food is powerful!

Everything you're learning here? This is what Stephanie's nutritionist taught her. As she started to understand the relationship between her symptoms and her food choices, Stephanie was able to make small, incremental adjustments in the right direction.

You can do the same.

APPROACHES TO ANTI-INFLAMMATORY EATING

Fortunately, making anti-inflammatory, pro–mental health choices doesn't necessarily mean giving up everything else. It's more about balance, or nudging yourself in the right direction.

Often it's just a question of eating *more* of the good stuff. One study found that just eating more fruits and vegetables—without changing anything else—caused a substantial drop in inflammation levels. All the participants had to do was jump from eating two servings of fruits and vegetables a day to eating eight servings. They got the benefits in just four weeks, without having to give anything up.[44]

To be honest, that's the kind of study I love because it makes me think, *This is actually something I can do.* It's manageable.

There are far too many studies about food and inflammation to cite them all here. The upshot is that the same diets that have been proven to improve overall health and longevity, or reduce the risk of disease, almost always have one key thing in common: their effects on inflammation.

Short version: they are all rich in foods that have anti-inflammatory effects in the body and brain, and they avoid foods that promote inflammation.

---

44 Bernhard Watzl et al., "A 4-Wk Intervention with High Intake of Carotenoid-Rich Vegetables and Fruit Reduces Plasma C-Reactive Protein in Healthy, Nonsmoking Men," *American Journal of Clinical Nutrition* 82, no. 5 (November 2005): 1052–58, https://doi.org/10.1093/ajcn/82.5.1052.

All this theoretical knowledge is great. But what should you actually put on your shopping list? What should you actually eat? Or not eat? Take breakfast, for example. Should you pick blueberries or bacon? With blueberries, you're starting your day on a high note, heading down a path to lower inflammation. The bacon, unfortunately, goes the other way. No matter how tasty bacon is, choosing the blueberries means choosing your mental health.

In general, anti-inflammatory foods are fresh, whole, and plant-based. They include fresh fruits and vegetables, nuts and seeds, and leafy greens. And also cold-water fish, like salmon and sardines, that are rich in healthy fats.

On the flip side, pro-inflammatory foods tend to be processed, preserved, animal based, and sugar loaded. Think packaged cookies and fast food. Unfortunately, these kinds of foods make up a large part of many people's diets.

I've put together the list below to show you some foods to consider adding to your grocery list, as well as some to buy a little less frequently. What I've included here are the most powerful and evidence-supported anti-inflammatory foods and some of the more common and potentially damaging pro-inflammatory ones.

Remember how I told you to focus on small wins? Here's one: if you can tip the balance of your shopping list even a little bit toward the anti-inflammatory side of this list, you'll already be on the road to reducing your symptoms and improving your quality of life.

WHAT TO ADD TO YOUR SHOPPING LIST
(THE ANTI-INFLAMMATORY FOODS)

Blueberries	Leafy Greens	Avocados	Beans/Legumes
Chia Seeds	Cherry Tomatoes	Green Tea	Broccoli
Whole grains	Ground Flax	Olive Oil	Almonds
Walnuts	Salmon	Sesame Oil	Oranges
Ginger	Garlic	Turmeric	Cherries
Kombucha	Sauerkraut[45]		

WHAT TO LEAVE OFF YOUR SHOPPING LIST
(THE MOST PRO-INFLAMMATORY FOODS)

Cookies	French Fries	Candy	Hot Dogs
Sodas	Sausage	Hamburgers	Margarine
Potato Chips	Pastries	Crackers	Creamy Dressings

NOT SO SWEET: SUGAR AND INFLAMMATION

I'm afraid I've got some bad news for you. Sugar isn't your friend when it comes to inflammation.

It's really tough to cut down on sugar because our bodies crave it. Before modern food production made sugar easily available, sugar was hard to find, and there wasn't much to go around. Whenever early humans found some—in fruit or honey, usually—they would eat as much as they could.

---

45 Roma Pahwa, Amandeep Goyal, and Ishwarlal Jialal, *Chronic Inflammation* (Treasure Island, FL: StatPearls Publishing, 2018), https://www.ncbi.nlm.nih.gov/books/NBK493173/.

Now, though, we have access to all the sugar we want, all the time. It's everywhere: pastries, candy, sweetened beverages like soda and energy drinks. Modern foods contain more sugar than our bodies can handle.

Unfortunately, sugar is a key factor in chronic inflammation and auto-immune diseases, including multiple sclerosis, arthritis, skin conditions, and inflammatory bowel disease.[46] And cutting down on your sugar intake reduces risk factors for all kinds of chronic diseases, including inflammation.[47]

In other words, removing even some of the sugar from your diet can be one of the most important actions you take for your own mental health.

SCIENCE-PROVEN FUEL STRATEGIES

The key takeaway from this chapter is that getting more anti-inflammatory foods and fewer pro-inflammatory ones will improve your mental health. But it is easier to make good choices if you have the specifics, so I'll show you a couple of common approaches. The ones I've outlined here aren't requirements or strict regimens. They're also not "diets" in the traditional sense. They are evidence-backed strategies for introducing more good stuff and getting the benefits of anti-inflammatory eating.

Think of these as delicious options to add to your anti-inflammatory tool kit.

---

46 Xiao Ma et al., "Excessive Intake of Sugar: An Accomplice of Inflammation," *Frontiers in Immunology* 13 (2022), https://doi.org/10.3389/fimmu.2022.988481.

47 Kerrie A. Hart et al., "Decreased Consumption of Sugar-Sweetened Beverages Improved Selected Biomarkers of Chronic Disease Risk among US Adults: 1999 to 2010," *Nutrition Research* 34, no. 1 (January 2014): 58–65, https://doi.org/10.1016/j.nutres.2013.10.005.

MEDITERRANEAN DIET

Imagine a sun-drenched patio with the sea rolling in the background. On the patio is a table, piled high with fresh salads, whole grains, bowls of nuts and seeds, and glittering bottles of just-squeezed olive oil. There's a platter of salmon at one end, a dish with bright red tomatoes and crisp green cucumbers, and a steaming pot of five-bean soup. You just imagined the basics of the Mediterranean Diet. Doesn't sound too bad, does it?

One of the things I think people forget about anti-inflammatory eating is that it doesn't have to be restrictive or flavorless. The truth is, anti-inflammatory foods tend to be the ones our bodies were designed to eat: fresh fruits and vegetables, nuts and seeds, and other natural and delicious options.

The Mediterranean Diet is one of the best-studied approaches to anti-inflammatory eating. Back in the 1950s, researchers noticed that people who lived in the areas surrounding the Mediterranean Sea had amazing health outcomes. They had lower rates of heart disease and cancer and longer, healthier lives overall.

The traditional, plant-based foods they ate contributed powerfully to their long-term health. Although they didn't know it at the time, the anti-inflammatory properties of those foods played a critical role. As one recent meta-analysis of all the existing studies on the Mediterranean Diet put it, "The majority of beneficial effects could be primarily related to its anti-inflammatory and antioxidant properties."[48]

There are plenty of Mediterranean cookbooks out there, if you need help getting started, but the critical points are fresh-plant foods and the produce of the Mediterranean, including tomatoes, garlic, olive oil, beans, and leafy greens.

---

48   Mauro Finicelli et al., "The Mediterranean Diet: An Update of the Clinical Trials," *Nutrients* 14, no. 14 (July 19, 2022): 2956, https://doi.org/10.3390/nu14142956.

DASH

DASH, or Dietary Approaches to Stop Hypertension, is similar to the Mediterranean Diet but was specifically designed to help people lower their blood pressure. The DASH diet includes foods that are rich in vitamins and minerals, low in red meat and sugar, and focused on fresh, whole-plant foods.

And guess what? It turns out that what's good for the heart is good for the brain.

The DASH diet was designed to reduce the risk of heart disease, but it also lowers inflammation and improves brain health.[49] A 2023 study conducted by researchers at Harvard Medical School found that people on the DASH diet lowered their levels of several inflammation markers, including the major player C-reactive protein, by almost 20 percent in just 12 weeks, compared to a group of people eating a "typical American Diet" which actually *increased* their inflammation in the same period of time.[50]

Like I said before: every system in your body is connected. What's good for your heart is also good for your brain.

A DIET SPECIALLY MADE FOR YOUR MIND?

Researchers have combined the best insights from research studies (and the DASH and Mediterranean diets) to create the MIND approach: a fuel strategy specifically created for brain health. And it's super easy. Just put together the recommended foods, like berries, nuts, and beans, into whatever meals you want.

If that doesn't get you excited, maybe these research findings will:

---

49 Stephen P. Jurashek et al., "Effects of Diet and Sodium Reduction on Cardiac Injury, Strain, and Inflammation: The DASH-Sodium Trial," *Journal of the American College of Cardiology* 77, no. 21 (June 2021): 2625–34, https://doi.org/10.1016/j.jacc.2021.03.320.

50 Sepideh Soltani, Maryam J. Chitsazi, and Amin Salehi-Abargouei, "The Effect of Dietary Approaches to Stop Hypertension (DASH) on Serum Inflammatory Markers: A Systematic Review and Meta-Analysis of Randomized Trials," *Clinical Nutrition* 37, no. 2 (April 2018): 542–50, https://doi.org/10.1016/j.clnu.2017.02.018.

- Several large studies have shown that the MIND diet participants had better cognitive functioning, larger total brain volume, higher memory scores, lower risk of dementia, and slower cognitive decline, even when the studies included participants with Alzheimer's disease and history of stroke.[51]
- A randomized controlled trial found that the MIND diet can reverse the negative effects of obesity on cognition and brain structure.[52] Not prevent. Not stop the damage from continuing. Actually *reverse* it.

I always get excited when I see tangible ways to improve brain health like this, especially when it's within easy reach in my own life.

KETO

I can't tell you how many people have asked me about the ketogenic, or "keto," diet. "Going keto" has gotten a ton of press recently because it's endorsed by a lot of athletes and celebrities. Basically, keto minimizes carbohydrates (carbs) and focuses instead on healthy fats and proteins. Carbohydrates are digested into sugar molecules, and they're found in everything from bread and pasta to potatoes and corn.

Our early ancestors had far fewer reliable food sources than we do, and they often had to go long periods without access to fruits and grains. As a result, our bodies evolved to respond to carbohydrate shortages by burning fat and other molecules instead of sugar. Keto restricts carb intake to switch your body over into this fat-burning mode. The shift creates the keto benefits you've probably heard of, like appetite suppression and increased energy.

---

51 Harvard T. H. Chan School of Public Health, "Diet Review: MIND Diet," *The Nutrition Source* (blog), last reviewed August 2023, https://www.hsph.harvard.edu/nutritionsource/healthy-weight/diet-reviews/mind-diet/.

52 Golnaz Arjmand, Mojtaba Abbas-Zadeh, and Mohammad Hassan Eftekhari, "Effect of MIND Diet Intervention on Cognitive Performance and Brain Structure in Healthy Obese Women: A Randomized Controlled Trial," *Scientific Reports* 12 (February 21, 2022): 2871, https://doi.org/10.1038/s41598-021-04258-9.

But the keto diet has something that a lot of other celebrity-endorsed fads don't have. Science.

Many studies have shown that a ketogenic diet reduces inflammation in conditions from arthritis to chronic pain.[53] Remember in Chapter Three when we talked about free radicals? Keto helps knock them out too.[54]

One study even showed that a keto diet can turn off the activity of some pro-inflammatory genes.[55]

WHAT'S A KETONE?

Whenever I hear the word *ketone* (pronounced key-tone), I always think of jazz bands, like "Dietary Fiber and the Ketones" or something. Actually, ketones are chemicals made in your liver. When you substantially reduce carbohydrate intake, like you do on the keto diet, your body converts fats into ketones, which provide an alternate energy source in your body.

Ketones turn out to have an anti-inflammatory effect in the body and brain.[56] And having even slightly higher levels of ketones in the blood

---

53 Salman A. Alhamzah, Othman M. Gatar, and Nawaf W. Alruwaili, "Effects of Ketogenic Diet on Oxidative Stress and Cancer: A Literature Review," *Advances in Cancer Biology–Metastasis* 7 (July 2023): 100093, https://doi.org/10.1016/j.adcanc.2023.100093; and Rowena Field, Fereshteh Pourkazemi, and Kieron Rooney, "Effects of a Low-Carbohydrate Ketogenic Diet on Reported Pain, Blood Biomarkers and Quality of Life in Patients with Chronic Pain: A Pilot Randomized Clinical Trial," *Pain Medicine* 23, no. 2 (February 2022): 326–38, https://doi.org/10.1093/pm/pnab278.

54 Alessandro Pinto et al., "Anti-Oxidant and Anti-Inflammatory Activity of Ketogenic Diet: New Perspectives for Neuroprotection in Alzheimer's Disease," *Antioxidants* 7, no. 5 (April 28, 2018): 63, https://doi.org/10.3390/antiox7050063.

55 Markus Bock, Mirjam Karber, and Hartmut Kuhn, "Ketogenic Diets Attenuate Cyclooxygenase and Lipoxygenase Gene Expression in Multiple Sclerosis," *eBioMedicine* 36 (October 2018): 293–303, https://doi.org/10.1016/j.ebiom.2018.08.057.

56 Yun-Hee Youm et al., "The Ketone Metabolite β-Hydroxybutyrate Blocks NLRP3 Inflammasome-Mediated Inflammatory Disease," *Nature Medicine* 21 (March 2015): 263–69, https://doi.org/10.1038/nm.3804; and Rita Polito et al., "The Ketogenic Diet and Neuroinflammation: The Action of Beta-Hydroxybutyrate in a Microglial Cell Line," *International Journal of Molecular Science* 24, no. 4 (February 4, 2023): 3102, https://doi.org/10.3390/ijms24043102.

(one result of the keto diet) can reduce cardiac inflammation and slow the development of heart failure.[57]

That's a lot of reward for giving up your breakfast pastries.

Even though it can seem like a fad, the keto diet has actually been around for more than 100 years. It was first developed in the Mayo Clinic in the 1920s by a doctor named Russell Wilder. Wilder was trying to find ways to help children with severe seizure disorders. In some cases, these people had multiple seizures per day, making it almost impossible for them to manage their lives. Up to that time, their conditions had been untreatable.

Wilder believed that ketones could help, and amazingly, it worked.[58]

The development of effective anti-seizure drugs means that the keto diet has been used less often for seizure disorders. But in the 1990s, keto reemerged as a method for improving general health.

Because of its neuroprotective effect, keto is now offered as a complementary treatment not only for epilepsy but also for Alzheimer's disease.[59] It's also showing promise as a preventative measure—and possibly even a therapy—for some cancers.[60]

The downside? It's very hard to stick to and do well. A lot of people have strong cravings and end up eating a diet of bacon and cheese (which can cause other health problems) instead of the healthier version based on leafy greens and plant-based oils.

But for those who are willing to make substantial changes in how

57 Nikole J. Byrne et al., "Chronically Elevating Circulating Ketones Can Reduce Cardiac Inflammation and Blunt the Development of Heart Failure," *Circulation: Heart Failure* 13, no. 6 (June 4, 2020): e006573, https://doi.org/10.1161/circheartfailure.119.006573.

58 Jae-Moon Kim, "Ketogenic Diet: Old Treatment, New Beginning," *Clinical Neurophysiology Practice* 2 (2017): 161–62, https://doi.org/10.1016/j.cnp.2017.07.001.

59 Pinto et al., "Anti-Oxidant and Anti-Inflammatory Activity of Ketogenic Diet."

60 Alhamzah, Gatar, and Alruwaili, "Effects of a Ketogenic Diet on Oxidative Stress and Cancer."

they eat, reducing carbohydrates and getting energy from fats and proteins instead can be life-changing.

INTERMITTENT FASTING

"Fasting" makes a lot of people think of monks on mountaintops not eating for weeks, or boxers going without food for days to make their weight class. It can come across as too weird or too difficult to apply to normal life.

In fact, fasting is less about not eating and more about *when* you eat. You already fast to some extent every day. If you eat dinner at 7:00 p.m. and then don't get around to having breakfast until 10:00 a.m. the next morning, congratulations! You were fasting during that whole time.

Think about intermittent fasting not as choosing not to eat, but as choosing only to eat during certain hours. For example, you might decide that you will eat between the hours of 1:00 p.m. and 8:00 p.m. every day.

Why would you do this? Because longer periods between eating switches your body into non-digesting mode. If you've eaten recently, your body tends to use sugars for energy because they are easily available. It's hard work to convert fats and proteins to energy, so your body uses sugars instead.

A few hours after eating, though, your body switches over. There aren't as many sugars available, so the body starts burning fat instead.

To get the maximum benefits from this switch, you have to stretch out the period of time between meals. You can do that by only eating during certain times of day, or you can try only eating one meal a couple of days a week. How you do it doesn't matter as much as sticking to a routine and giving your body a chance to switch regularly.

Researchers found that fasting reduces inflammation and improves chronic inflammatory diseases. And better yet, it does this without affecting the immune system's ability to respond to infections.[61] In

---

61 Stefan Jordan et al., "Dietary Intake Regulates the Circulating Inflammatory Monocyte Pool," *Cell* 178, no. 5 (August 22, 2019): 1102–114, https://doi.org/10.1016/j.cell.2019.07.050.

other words, you don't have to worry that fasting will "weaken" you or make you more susceptible to other conditions.

One fascinating study found that people who fast for Ramadan—the "holy month" in which Muslims fast all day and focus on spiritual growth—had reduced inflammatory markers, as well as lower body-fat percentage (among other health benefits).[62] It's kind of incredible to think that so many spiritual traditions figured out the mental and personal benefits of fasting long before research could show us why it works.

One caution though. You should definitely consult with a doctor before starting a fasting diet—and monitor your feelings of hunger so that the fasting doesn't become a source of stress in itself. Also, if fasting is a trigger for any of your mental health issues (such as disordered eating), it's especially important to talk to a healthcare provider before starting.

Mental Health Benefits, Direct from Your Kitchen Sink

This chapter is mostly about food, but I would be remiss not to talk about another vital and accessible tool for repairing mental health: water.

Nothing in your mind or body works properly without enough water. Dehydration reduces executive function (activities like planning, remembering, and juggling tasks) and attention, and one two-year study found that people who were chronically dehydrated had decreased cognitive performance.[63]

Even mild dehydration has been shown to affect focus and mood

---

62 Mo'ez Al-Islam E. Faris et al., "Intermittent Fasting during Ramadan Attenuates Proinflammatory Cytokines and Immune Cells in Healthy Subjects," *Nutrition Research* 32, no. 12 (December 2012): 947–55, https://doi.org/10.1016/j.nutres.2012.06.021.

63 Matthew T. Wittbrodt and Melinda Millard-Stafford, "Dehydration Impairs Cognitive Performance: A Meta-Analysis," *Medicine & Science in Sports & Exercise* 50, no. 11 (November 2018): 2360–68, https://doi.org/10.1249/mss.0000000000001682; and Stephanie K. Nishi et al., "Water Intake, Hydration Status and 2-Year Changes in Cognitive Performance: A Prospective Cohort Study," *BMC Medicine* 21 (March 2023): 82, https://doi.org/10.1186/s12916-023-02771-4.

in otherwise healthy women, leading to reduced vigor, higher fatigue, less ability to concentrate, higher perception of task difficulty, and greater likelihood of developing headaches.[64] Mild dehydration also reduces cognitive ability and mood in otherwise healthy men, including increases in tension and anxiety, a greater likelihood of errors, and increased fatigue.[65] For most people struggling with any mental health issues, these are likely to be very familiar symptoms.

And water matters beyond everyday quality of life as well. Studies have found that people over age 65 who are dehydrated have a higher risk of dementia—and in a tragic cycle, people with dementia are more likely to be dehydrated.[66]

Because you can't do fancy molecular analysis at home to find out whether you're officially dehydrated, it can be hard to figure out how much water is enough. The key is to listen to your body. If you're getting fatigued or having trouble concentrating, ask yourself if you've been drinking water. Also, keep water near you throughout the day and get in the habit of drinking some regularly.

What are you waiting for? Go get some water! I'll be right here.

RECOMMENDATIONS

Remember what I promised at the beginning of this chapter? Simple solutions. Small wins. Minimum effort for maximum impact.

Where fuel is concerned, tipping the balance a little each day is the key.

So first, take a look at your grocery list and compare it to the one earlier in this chapter (it is based on the MIND approach). Can

---

64 Lawrence E. Armstrong et al., "Mild Dehydration Affects Mood in Healthy Young Women," *Journal of Nutrition* 142, no. 2 (February 2012): 382–88, https://doi.org/10.3945/jn.111.142000.

65 Matthew S. Ganio et al., "Mild Dehydration Impairs Cognitive Performance and Mood of Men," *British Journal of Nutrition* 106, no. 10 (2011): 1535–43, https://doi.org/10.1017/s0007114511002005.

66 Michele Lauriola et al., "Neurocognitive Disorders and Dehydration in Older Patients: Clinical Experience Supports the Hydromolecular Hypothesis of Dementia," *Nutrients* 10, no. 5 (May 3, 2018): 562, https://doi.org/10.3390/nu10050562.

you replace potato chips with berries? Could you think about throwing a few "Mediterranean" foods, like fresh tomatoes or dark leafy greens, into your basket? Maybe replace a sugary drink with hot tea or water?

Switch out one or two items a week and see how you feel. Every little change makes a difference.

Once you've got a bit more of the good stuff (and hopefully a bit less of the pro-inflammatory stuff) on your list, it might be time to think about *when* you eat, and how often. Could you extend the time between dinner and breakfast a little more? Could you skip breakfast one day this week?

Food should be fuel, helping your body and mind stay healthy and well. Unfortunately, the food we eat as a culture tends to be a stressor instead, causing and increasing inflammation rather than fighting it. Trying to force yourself onto a restrictive diet can feel like it's increasing that stress. As a result, shifting your food choices can seem like a lot to ask.

But it doesn't have to be.

Add just a few more bites of anti-inflammatory foods each day and reduce your intake of pro-inflammatory foods. These small changes will start to rebalance your system, creating the foundation you need to repair your brain and rebuild your mental health. And grab a glass of water when you do!

Food can either improve your mental health, or it can be another stressor. You can choose.

FUEL BETTER, FEEL BETTER

Stephanie discovered the power of small changes for herself.

When she found out she'd developed celiac disease, she set up an appointment with a nutritionist. The nutritionist helped her review her food choices. Even though Stephanie tried to make healthy food for her family, she realized she'd been eating a lot more "comfort foods" recently to help her cope with her panic attacks and her busy schedule.

Unfortunately for her, most of those comfort foods contained wheat, which triggered her celiac problems. And all of them were pro-inflammatory, meaning that they were also contributing to the inflammation cycle that, in turn, contributed to her symptoms.

She and her nutritionist worked together to replace those foods with anti-inflammatory options that wouldn't irritate her bowel. Every day, Stephanie ate a few more of the new foods and cut out a few of the old ones.

Even after just a month, the relief was incredible. Where she used to have cramps that laid her out on the couch every couple of days, now they only happened every couple of weeks. Her brain felt clearer. She was less anxious about food and getting to the bathroom.

Less stomach pain also meant better sleep. For the first time in more than a year, she got several nights of continuous sleep without being woken up by pain and cramping. Every morning, she felt a little better.

Maybe best of all, she didn't have to plan her days around being close to a bathroom at all times. She could start coaching her kids' games again.

She still parks down the street from the school. Driving still causes her heart rate to skyrocket. Her PTSD isn't gone, and she knows she'll need to seek out other help to solve that problem. But for the first time in years, she feels like she might actually have the energy to take that on.

Putting the right fuel into your body is critical for physical and mental health, but you also need to get that fuel where it needs to go. That's where movement comes in.

So go grab a healthy snack and get ready to hop, skip, and jump—or at least stand, stretch, and walk—to better brain health.

TL;DR

→ Food is fuel for the brain as well as the body. Giving your brain and body good quality fuel can have a powerful impact on chronic inflammation and brain health.

→ Small adjustments, like eating more of the anti-inflammatory foods listed in this chapter and fewer of the pro-inflammatory ones, can have big effects over time. Remember that eating a few extra servings of fruit and vegetables (without changing anything else) can drop inflammation levels in just four weeks!

→ If you find it easier to follow nutrition plans with a structure, you're in luck! There are well-researched options like MIND, Mediterranean, and DASH—take a look at each and see what suits you best.

→ When and how you eat can also make a difference. Intermittent fasting in particular has been shown to significantly reduce inflammation and inflammation-related symptoms and disorders.

CHAPTER FIVE

MOVE YOUR BODY, DE-STRESS YOUR MIND

As a kid, Camilla was always active. She remembers running around the playground with her friends, playing hard and moving freely. But then the pain started. Over the years, as the pain got worse, she avoided physical activity more. Now she can't remember the last time she took a long walk, much less ran or danced.

She's never really liked gyms either. All the noise. The people wrapped up in their own worlds inside their headphones, loudly dropping weights or sprinting on the treadmill. She's never felt comfortable in that environment.

Now, though, she's thinking about how she might get moving again.

During her most recent medical checkup, her naturopath gave her some interesting information. They'd just gotten back from a conference, where they learned that exercise could reduce exactly the kinds of symptoms Camilla is struggling with most.

Camilla was concerned. What about her pain? Her fatigue? Shouldn't she be taking it easy?

But her naturopath assured her she didn't have to run 20 miles or do a high-intensity cardio class.

"Why not start out with something low-impact and see how you feel?" they asked.

One thing they learned at the conference, they told Camilla, was that physical activity doesn't have to be strenuous or sweaty to be effective. Camilla wouldn't have to go to a gym if she didn't want to, and she didn't have to do anything that would hurt.

Still a bit apprehensive, Camilla talked through some options with them, but she was worried. She's already in pain a lot of the time. Wouldn't exercise make it even worse?

"Camilla, your pain is getting worse now, and your fatigue is so bad you can barely see clients. If an hour of moving your body in a pool feels good, you haven't lost anything. And if it helps, it could make a big difference in your day-to-day experience."

After a few other options, the naturopath mentioned water aerobics. Camilla agreed to look up the website for the local pool, and on the way home, she decided she might as well sign up for a class.

MADE TO MOVE

Camilla's experience is so familiar to me. All the time, people come to our brain fitness centers with pain and fatigue, wondering whether physical activity will help or hurt. Just like Camilla, many of them wonder if exercise could make their pain worse or overstress their already-exhausted bodies.

This chapter answers those questions and offers some steps that you can take to get moving toward better brain health.

For myself, I have to say: I love moving. I love being active. I love throwing a frisbee outside with friends and chasing kids around a backyard BBQ.

But as much as I love moving, I absolutely hate being told to "exercise." Exercise sounds like hard work. It sounds repetitive. It sounds like my high school swim coach yelling at me to keep pace.

Exercise reminds me of feeling bad about the gym membership I'm not using enough and cursing the alarm clock that's telling me I "should" get up and work out.

Exercise is what everybody is constantly telling us to do more of, while we avoid it using whatever excuse we can.

All I can say is, *ugh*. No, thanks.

That's why I promise not to talk about exercise in this chapter. Instead, I want to talk about movement.

Your body is made to move. It needs to move.

Just like with food, I'm going to give you the min/max on movement. And just like with food, the key takeaway is simple: any additional movement is a positive step toward reducing inflammation.

If you love the elliptical in your gym, more power to you. But you don't need machines, programs, or memberships to get the critical anti-inflammatory benefits of movement.

In fact, let's take a second to talk about some common myths about movement. (Although to be fair, most of these myths are really about exercise!)

BUSTING MOVEMENT MYTHS

Myth: You have to push yourself as hard as you can.

Reality: Increasing your movement until you're breathing a bit harder or feeling warm is enough to get the main benefits. Movement for mental health is about getting your blood moving, getting oxygen and nutrients to every part of your body. You don't have to push yourself to your limits to get there. Lighter exercise can give your brain what it needs to be protected from stress.[67]

---

67 Hideaki Soya et al., "BDNF Induction with Mild Exercise in the Rat Hippocampus," *Biochemical and Biophysical Research Communications* 358, no. 4 (July 2007): 961–67, https://doi.org/10.1016/j. bbrc.2007.04.173.

Myth: You have to exercise every day to get benefits.

Reality: You don't. With exercise, more isn't always better. One study that compared two groups of people with drug-resistant depression found that the group that did just 25 percent as much exercise as the other group got the same benefits.[68] A little bit goes a long way.

Myth: You have to be sweating like crazy for it to count.

Reality: Nope. This one is very similar to the first myth, but it's important to call it out separately. Working up a sweat can feel great. Intense activity can be good for you. But you don't have to be sweating to get the anti-inflammatory, stress-reducing, healthy benefits of movement.

Myth: You have to be exhausted afterward to get benefits.

Reality: All movement is beneficial. In fact, any additional time spent *not sitting* is beneficial, no matter what else you're doing. You don't have to be huffing and puffing. You don't have to put aside two hours to really "wear yourself out." Just move. When you're chronically stressed, intense exercise can actually be a bad thing, so the key is to move, not to strain yourself.[69]

I hope you're starting to see a pattern here.

All movement is good movement. It doesn't have to be hard, punishing, or extreme to reduce inflammation and stress and improve your quality of life.

Actually—let's try something. If you're sitting on the couch or at

---

68   Chad D. Rethorst et al., "Pro-Inflammatory Cytokines as Predictors of Antidepressant Effects of Exercise in Major Depressive Disorder," *Molecular Psychiatry* 18, (2013): 1119–24, https://doi.org/10.1038%2Fmp.2012.125.

69   Érica Cerqueira et al., "Inflammatory Effects of High and Moderate Intensity Exercise—A Systematic Review," *Frontiers of Physiology* 10 (2019), https://doi.org/10.3389/fphys.2019.01550.

your table or desk reading this book, put it down for one minute, stand up, stretch a bit, and move your legs. Maybe take a walk around the living room or up and down the stairs. I'll wait.

Are you back? Great. That was movement. It counts! Every time you move, that's a win.

I think you're getting the point. Any additional movement is healthy, and most of the benefits of movement aren't visible in terms of sweat, bulging muscles, huffing and puffing, or looking great in yoga pants.

The benefits that matter, the benefits we're going to focus on in this chapter, are the ones you can't see: decreases in inflammation and improvements in your mental health. That's what this is all about.

BLOOD FLOW MATTERS

You know the guy at the gym who makes all that noise lifting 300-pound weights? That guy is hoping to get a very specific benefit. He is building his muscles to create a particular body shape. (He might also be hoping that the cute personal trainer across the gym notices him, but that's another story.)

What about your neighbor who gets up every morning and runs 20 miles before work? She's also got specific goals in mind. Maybe she's trying to win a marathon or get on *American Ninja Warrior*.

The point is, people *exercise* for a lot of different reasons, from medaling in the Olympics to impressing their old classmates at the next high school reunion.

If those are your goals, that's great. But we're not concerned with any of that. What we're concerned with is blood flow. That's why our focus is on *moving*.

Blood flow, or circulation, is necessary for life. If eating well is about getting the building blocks your cells need into your system, circulation is about distributing those building blocks to the cells themselves through the blood vessels.

Often, we think of blood vessels as only carrying blood cells, but that's not quite true. Red blood cells do make up part of the blood.

Red blood cells carry oxygen throughout the body, and they are the reason we think of blood as red. But the blood vessels also act as a transport system for all kinds of other cargo.

When your immune system triggers the release of white blood cells, they are carried through the blood vessels. When your glands release hormones, they release them into the bloodstream to be carried where they are needed. The blood vessels also transport nutrients like glucose, fats, and proteins. Even disease agents like flu viruses travel through the bloodstream. And when cells are damaged or die, their waste products can end up in the bloodstream as well.

Essentially, your circulatory system is the transportation system for everything that goes out to, and comes back from, every cell in your body.

If your body were a forest, the bloodstream would be the streams and lakes and rivers, bringing water and nutrients to the trees and plants so they could thrive. There are big, wide, rushing rivers and small streams—and even tiny rivulets running through the soil when it rains. Your bloodstream is the same way, flowing from wide, high-volume vessels near the middle of your body out to smaller and smaller vessels in your extremities and organs.

And just like the forest becomes stressed (and more susceptible to fires) when its water-feeding systems dry up, your body's stress increases when nutrients and immune responders and other important health-and-repair molecules can't reach your cells.

That goes double for your brain. I've said it before, and I'll probably say it again: your brain only takes up about 2 percent of your body weight, but it uses 20 percent of your energy. That's because it's running everything from your heartbeat to your job performance. Getting nutrients and oxygen to every part of your body is important, but getting them to your brain is critical.

Movement pushes your heart rate up, opens your blood vessels, and increases circulation in your brain. It's kind of like widening a canal to let more nutrient-rich water flow into a downstream ecosystem. When you move, blood moves, carrying with it everything your cells need to be healthy. You experience lower stress and feel better, and the inflammation response is calmed.

SEDENTARY LIFESTYLE: A DAM IN THE RIVER

A sedentary lifestyle, without regular movement, keeps the blood from getting where it needs to go. Even if you're putting all the right nutrients into your body, they can't do any good if they aren't getting to the cells and organs where they're needed.

Not moving is like putting a dam across your body's nutrient streams. If you're in the same seated position for ten hours a day, blood isn't flowing properly. It's getting pooled in some areas and not reaching others. It's not moving around. Over time, this lack of movement causes damage across the entire body-brain system in the form of chronic disease.

I think one group of researchers put it best when they said that our modern, sedentary lifestyle "appears to have dire health consequences."[70] Yikes.

Oh, and those researchers also found that the link between inactivity and chronic disease was...you guessed it...inflammation.

THE INFLAMMATION CONNECTION

So you already know that chronic inflammation cuts off the nutrient and oxygen supply to your cells. Over time, if it occurs too much or for too long, this kind of constriction can create a tourniquet-like effect and reduce cell functioning wherever it occurs.

Most importantly for mental health, this effect also occurs in the brain, and constricted blood flow in the brain can damage or kill neurons. Like all other cells, neurons need oxygen and fuel to

---

70 Roberto Carlos Burini et al., "Inflammation, Physical Activity, and Chronic Disease: An Evolutionary Perspective," *Sports Medicine and Health Science* 2, no. 1 (March 2020): 1–6, https://doi.org/10.1016/j.smhs.2020.03.004.

function. When the blood vessels that feed them are impacted by inflammation, the neurons struggle to survive. As we know, the brain has all kinds of mechanisms to heal and repair itself. But low nutrient and oxygen supplies reduce that capacity for self-repair. The chronic inflammation cycle sets in.

Symptoms like fatigue, brain fog, anxiety, and depression can be the result.

Movement brings needed nutrients and repair mechanisms to cells and reduces the physical stress experienced by your body. Repeated, long-term studies show that movement reduces inflammation, substantially increases the functioning of the body's repair systems, and dramatically improves mental health. No wonder movement is shown to be at least as effective against depression as any of the currently available medications.[71]

What makes movement even more powerful is that it reduces inflammation (or even reverses its effects) through multiple different pathways. In other words, movement doesn't have just one positive impact on the body. It has many overlapping effects that are beneficial separately and even more beneficial in combination.

Let's break that down for a minute by looking at depression specifically. It's well-proven at this point that inflammation can both cause and worsen depression. What researchers have discovered is that it does this through a number of different pathways. It disrupts the work of neurotransmitters in your brain, it alters the function of the HPA axis (the hormone-balancing system we talked about in Chapter Three), and it increases pro-inflammatory processes in the brain and body.

That's one reason depression is so hard to treat: it's coming at you from many body systems at once.

Guess what? *Movement impacts every single one of those pathways.*

---

71 Ben Singh et al., "Effectiveness of Physical Activity Interventions for Improving Depression, Anxiety and Distress: An Overview of Systematic Reviews," *British Journal of Sports Medicine* 57 (September 2023): 1203–209, https://doi.org/10.1136/bjsports-2022-106195.

That's worth saying again. Movement reduces inflammation by reversing or calming the effects in every one of the systems that are associated with depression and other mental health issues.[72]

My favorite thing about movement is that it has effects *now*. Not in six months. Not eventually. Now.

When you move, your blood vessels respond right away. The benefits start to happen as soon as your heart rate increases. So although there are incredible long-term benefits, including reducing chronic inflammation, movement also helps you feel better immediately.

For those of us struggling with mental health issues, having something that we can control, that can improve our symptoms right away, is life-changing.

INACTIVITY, INFLAMMATION, AND DEMENTIA

It's literally not possible to go into every study, and every piece of evidence, that links a sedentary lifestyle with poor brain health outcomes and inflammation. But I thought this one was too important to ignore: inactivity leads straight to dementia.[73]

To put it simply, sitting all the time causes damage to small blood vessels and decreases blood flow. Small blood vessel damage and decreased blood flow harms the white matter in your brain. Harm to the white matter in your brain speeds up cognitive decline.

Oof. That one hits me hard every time I think about it. We are really hurting ourselves by not moving enough.

72 Rethorst et al., "Pro-Inflammatory Cytokines as Predictors of Antidepressant Effects of Exercise."

73 Shijiao Yan et al., "Association between Sedentary Behavior and the Risk of Dementia: A Systematic Review and Meta-Analysis," *Translational Psychiatry* 10 (2020): 112, https://doi.org/10.1038% 2Fs41398-020-0799-5.

Like I said, I can't possibly cover every research link between inactivity and inflammation. Fortunately, somebody else did. If you want to know more about this specific connection, I highly recommend Jennifer Heisz's book *Move the Body, Heal the Mind*.

YOUR CLEANUP CREW

So here's kind of an odd thing we should address before we move on. While you're exercising, you are actually *increasing* stress on your body. Exercise itself, while you're doing it, is kind of, well, inflammatory. And yeah, I'll be using the word "exercise" for a bit here, because the kind of movement people think of as exercise—intense or high-impact movement—causes the biggest stress response.

But that doesn't always mean it's bad.

As long as it's not super-intense or excessively long, exercise creates only a mild form of stress—a form of stress your body is designed to handle. Exercise produces a small increase in inflammatory cytokines, as well as another form of messenger called *myokines*, which are specific to the muscles.[74]

They basically tell the body, "Hey, just FYI, we are out of our comfort zone here." This proactive inflammatory response compensates for the mild stress of exercise.

What's exciting is what happens next.

After you're done exercising, when your body gets the "back to normal" signal, it sends out a cleanup crew to clear out the inflammatory response it created. This cleanup crew is so effective that it also clears up additional inflammation that was there before the exercise even happened.[75]

---

74 Mai Charlotte Krogh Severinsen and Bente Klarlund Pedersen, "Muscle-Organ Crosstalk: The Emerging Roles of Myokines," *Endocrine Reviews* 41, no. 4 (August 2020): 594–609, https://doi.org/10.1210/endrev/bnaa016.

75 Michael Gleeson et al., "The Anti-Inflammatory Effects of Exercise: Mechanisms and Implications for the Prevention and Treatment of Disease," *Nature Reviews Immunology* 11 (August 2011): 607–615, https://doi.org/10.1038/nri3041.

It's like if you threw a party at your house. During the party, you might let dirty dishes pile up a bit more than normal and not sweep up after people tracking dirt in the house. The body's response to exercise is like a cleaning crew that shows up the next morning and is so good at their job, they don't just clean up from the party. They get your house cleaner than it was before!

This is one of the primary ways that exercise works to reduce overall inflammation, including the kinds of chronic inflammation that can damage your heart and depress your mood.[76] Strange as it sounds, the slight increase in inflammatory response during exercise creates an overall anti-inflammatory effect and even improves your cells' ability to heal themselves on their own.

FIXING YOUR STRESS "OFF" SWITCH

Exercise has another paradoxical effect: it reactivates your stress "off" switch.

When you're healthy, stress is a pretty short-lived, up-and-down cycle. You experience a stressor, the stress response comes online, and then (when the stressor goes away), your body flips the off switch. The stress response calms down, and you go back to baseline.

But as we talked about in Chapter Three, chronic stress damages your off switch. Instead of going through the quick up-and-down, you stay stuck in the "on" position. Over time, your body becomes numb to the stress response, and your body has to push hormones like cortisol really high for your cells to respond to them at all.

That puts you at constant, very high levels of stress hormones and damages the body and brain.

Exercise protects you from this effect by supplying a dose of BDNF (brain-derived neurotrophic factor). BDNF promotes growth and improves function and survival of brain cells—including the ones that turn off the stress response. Immediately after you exercise,

---

76 Gleeson et al., "The Anti-Inflammatory Effects of Exercise."

your brain is bathed in BDNF. Not only does it directly protect you from the damage caused by long-term inflammation, it reactivates the off switch.

It also downregulates, or lowers the production of, pro-inflammatory genes that have been associated with physical disease as well as mental health issues and suicide.[77] Some studies even suggest that BDNF might *prevent those genes from causing inflammation later, in subsequent stressful situations.*[78] What does that mean? It means that exercising today could help your body respond in less damaging ways when your boss is mad at you tomorrow or your kids are driving you nuts next week.

In other words, exercise helps protect against the damage caused by all the other stressors in your life—even ones you haven't experienced yet. And that's true even whether it's "exercise" or other forms of movement you might not think of that way.

One form of movement practice that can be especially effective at creating these positive effects is interval training.

STEP IT UP WITH INTERVALS

Most of us think of movement as something that we have to do for a long period of time, at least 20 or 30 minutes or more, to get the benefit. That's what movement scientists call "continuous" movement: you start moving and don't stop until you've met your time requirement.

Continuous movement is usually also *consistent* movement. In other words, you keep up the same approximate rate the whole time. If you jogged five miles, at about ten minutes per mile, that's

---

77   Cohen et al., "Chronic Stress, Glucocorticoid Receptor Resistance, Inflammation, and Disease Risk"; and Benoit Labonte et al., "Differential Glucocorticoid Receptor Exon 1_B, 1_C, and 1_H Expression and Methylation in Suicide Completers with a History of Childhood Abuse," *Biological Psychiatry* 72, no. 1 (July 1, 2012): 41–48, https://doi.org/10.1016/j.biopsych.2012.01.034.

78   Efthimia Kitraki, Despoina Karandrea, and Christos Kittas, "Long-Lasting Effects of Stress on Glucocorticoid Receptor Gene Expression in the Rat Brain," *Neuroendocrinology* 69, no. 5 (May 1999): 331–38, https://doi.org/10.1159/000054435.

continuous movement that's also consistent. That kind of movement gets your heart rate and blood flow up to a certain level and keeps them there.

Interval training is different. An "interval" is just a period of time when you change up the effort you're making. If you go for a walk in a hilly neighborhood, you'll notice yourself working a bit harder on the uphill, while the effort eases up on the downhill. Those are intervals of different effort.

Studies have found interval training to be beneficial in treating a bunch of inflammation-related diseases, including diabetes, Parkinson's, and rheumatoid arthritis, among others.[79] Recent research even suggests that while long, high-intensity movement bouts can increase some inflammation markers, interval training reduces them.[80]

It's that simple to incorporate interval training into your movement plan. You may have seen the term HIIT, or "high-intensity interval training," but what I'm talking about doesn't have to be nearly that intense; it's really just about varying your effort and working a little harder for short periods.

To give you a sense of just how accessible interval training can be, imagine you were part of this recent study. If you were in the control group, you'd just walk for ten minutes. If you got put in the interval training group, though, you would still walk for ten minutes—just at a varied pace. You'd walk slower for a few minutes, then pick it up to walk a bit faster, then slow down again. You'd repeat that pattern for the whole walk.

That's the whole thing.

79 José Manuel Leiva-Valderrama et al., "Effects of High-Intensity Interval Training on Inflammatory Biomarkers in Patients with Type 2 Diabetes. A Systematic Review," *International Journal of Environmental Research and Public Health* 18, no. 23 (November 30, 2021): 12644, https://doi. org/10.3390/ijerph182312644; Paulina Malczynska-Sims et al., "High-Intensity Interval Training Modulates Inflammatory Response in Parkinson's Disease," *Aging Clinical and Experimental Research* 34 (2022): 2165–76, https://doi.org/10.1007/s40520-022-02153-5; and David B. Bartlett et al., "Ten Weeks of High-Intensity Interval Walk Training Is Associated with Reduced Disease Activity and Improved Innate Immune Function in Older Adults with Rheumatoid Arthritis: A Pilot Study," *Arthritis Research & Therapy* 20 (June 14, 2018): 127, https://doi.org/10.1186/s13075-018-1624-x.

80 Malczynska-Sims et al., "High-Intensity Interval Training Modulates Inflammatory Response in Parkinson's Disease."

That small change—adding short periods of faster walking—-was the only difference between the groups. The interval group improved not only their fitness, but their memory as well, and both their health and memory gains were substantially higher than the gains in the consistent walking group. The interval training was good for their brains as well as their bodies.[81]

Interval training is easy to integrate into whatever movement you're already doing. When you go for a walk, pick up the pace a bit or find a few hills. You can even build intervals into your day-to-day routines. Try going up and down the stairs a couple times, walking around your living room, and going up and down the stairs again. It's that simple.

Or try this: every time you stand up and walk around, add in thirty seconds of jogging in place or lifting your knees up to your chest. Get your heart rate up, then back down, then up again for short periods of time. That's where you'll get your benefit. And you're likely to feel energized afterward, rather than worn out.

Whatever kind of movement you're already doing, you can throw in some intervals to increase its pro–mental health, anti-inflammatory effects.

As an added bonus, a lot of people I've worked with have found interval training a lot easier to start and to stick with than continuous, consistent movement.

Like I said: marathons not required!

RECOMMENDATIONS

The core message here is straightforward: as far as inflammation and mental health are concerned, any movement is good movement. Stand up and walk around. Swing your arms. Play with your kids or your grandkids. Stretch. Dance. Throw a ball for your dog.

Just move!

---

81   Ana Kovacevic et al., "The Effects of Aerobic Exercise Intensity on Memory in Older Adults," *Applied Physiology, Nutrition, and Metabolism* 45, no. 6 (June 2020): 591–600, https://doi.org/10.1139/apnm-2019-0495.

Movement that reduces inflammation and improves mental health doesn't have to be sweaty or grunty. It doesn't have to take place in the gym.

To get the benefits of movement right away, you really only need to remember one thing: get that heart rate up.

THE WORKOUT SWEET SPOT

So if it's important to get your heart rate up, how do you know you're doing it? And how do you know if you're getting it up enough to be beneficial?

The quick solution: take the talk test.

The talk test is just what it sounds like. You do it by talking while you're exercising. If you can talk normally and comfortably, just like you do when you're sitting down, you're probably not in the most beneficial heart rate zone. As soon as you find it a little harder to chat with your movement buddy, that's the sweet spot.

The talk test is based on a concept called the *lactate threshold*, and there's a bunch of science around it that you can look up if you want.[82] But the takeaway is that as soon as you're finding conversation harder than normal, you're in the zone.

THREE TIMES IS THE CHARM

Getting the full benefit of movement isn't just about intensity though. It's also about frequency: how often you're doing it.

Fortunately, researchers have looked into that as well. The amount of movement (or exercise) you need does depend on your goals. A professional soccer player, or someone who's training for a ski jump competition, probably needs frequent, high-intensity workouts.

---

82 Jennifer L. Reed and Andrew L. Pipe, "The Talk Test: A Useful Tool for Prescribing and Monitoring Exercise Intensity," *Current Opinion in Cardiology* 29, no. 5 (September 2014): 475–80, https://doi.org/10.1097/hco.0000000000000097.

But your goal is probably not to win the US Open. It's optimal mental health and quality of life—and the reduction of the stress-based and inflammation-driven symptoms that are making things hard for you now. That requires a different type, and frequency, of movement. One recent study that evaluated the effects of regular physical activity on people with high levels of anxiety found that the most effective schedule for improving and maintaining brain health was 30 minutes or so of light- to moderate-intensity movement three times a week.[83]

What does that really mean? Light to moderate intensity is the zone we were talking about earlier. You should get a little sweaty and warm, and it should be a bit harder to carry on a conversation. That's it. Do that, for half an hour, three times a week, and you will start getting the inflammation-fighting and mood-enhancing effects of movement for yourself. If you're feeling ambitious, throw in some intervals during that time to increase the benefit.

THE SITTING EPIDEMIC

We can't leave the movement chapter without addressing the other side of the picture: lack of movement. For a lot of us, the problem isn't just how much we should be exercising but how much time we spend sitting. Even if you spend time exercising, prolonged time sitting is still associated with poor health.[84]

When you sit, your body is crunched into the same position for hours at a time: legs bent, shoulders slumped, eyes forward. Your muscles get stiff, and you lose muscle tone. Let's be honest: I'm doing it right now.

83 K. M. Lucibello, J. Parker, and J. J. Heisz, "Examining a Training Effect on the State Anxiety Response to an Acute Bout of Exercise in Low and High Anxious Individuals," *Journal of Affective Disorders* 247 (March 15, 2019): 29–35, https://doi.org/10.1016/j.jad.2018.12.063.

84 Aviroop Biswas et al., "Sedentary Time and its Association with Risk for Disease Incidence, Mortality, and Hospitalization in Adults: A Systematic Review and Meta-Analysis," *Annals of Internal Medicine* 162, no. 2 (January 20, 2015): 123–32, https://doi.org/10.7326/M14-1651.

For most of us, there's no way to live our lives without periods of sitting. The question is, *how much sitting is too much?*

Sitting for long periods of time is so dangerous that the World Health Organization has identified sitting as a potential cause of cancer.[85] In older adults, higher amounts of sitting time are associated with higher mortality rates from inflammatory disease—even compared to people with low or moderate activity levels.[86]

In general, higher sitting times are associated with inflammatory disease, but also with insulin resistance and higher body mass index.[87]

While your three exercise sessions per week are really important, they don't necessarily keep you from sitting too much. You could sit ten hours a day and still get in your three workouts. To prevent the damage that comes from too much sitting, you need to move multiple times per day.

I don't mean you suddenly have to increase your workout frequency. The key here is just moving *some*, often. If you've been sitting for an hour, get up and walk around. Stretch. Take a minute to listen to some music and get the blood flowing. Then you can go right back to work if you need to.

One really good approach is just to set a timer for an hour. Every time it goes off, get up and move. It doesn't take long, you'll feel better and be able to concentrate more easily—and you'll be fighting inflammation all at the same time.

85 Fiona C. Bull et al., "World Health Organization 2020 Guidelines on Physical Activity and Sedentary Behaviour," *British Journal of Sports Medicine* 54, no. 24 (December 2020): 1451–62, https://doi.org/10.1136/bjsports-2020-102955.

86 Verónica Cabanas-Sánchez et al., "Physical Activity, Sitting Time, and Mortality from Inflammatory Diseases in Older Adults," *Frontiers in Physiology* 9 (July 11, 2018), https://doi.org/10.3389/fphys.2018.00898.

87 Thomas Yates et al., "Self-Reported Sitting Time and Markers of Inflammation, Insulin Resistance, and Adiposity," *American Journal of Preventive Medicine* 42, no. 1 (January 2012): 1–7, https://doi.org/10.1016/j.amepre.2011.09.022.

FEELING ALIVE AGAIN

Camilla's first water aerobics class was a nerve-racking experience. She woke up that morning in more pain than usual, and she was nervous about being the new person in the class. For a few moments, she considered canceling.

But then she remembered what her naturopath told her about the benefits, the possible pain relief, the better sleep—and she got up, packed her swim bag, and headed to the pool.

It's now been three months of regular classes, and she is so grateful she decided to go. Her pain isn't gone by any means, but it's much more manageable. Her body feels like her own again, able to move a bit more freely and get through the day with less fatigue.

The best part is the sense of vitality she's gotten back. It's like she's come back to life. She can look forward to things again. Maybe she'll even be able to travel to a professional training seminar she's been wanting to take.

She still has symptoms. She still has bad days—and some very bad days. But for the first time in a long time, she has something else: a small but growing belief that she might actually get better.

One of the benefits Camilla got from movement was better sleep. And that's an incredibly powerful benefit because sleep is one of the most important functions of the human body. Sleep heals. And as extreme as it sounds, not getting enough sleep can be deadly.

In the next chapter, I'll take you through the new research on the power of rest and show you how to use it to heal your brain and mind.

TL;DR

→ Your body needs movement to be healthy, and increasing the amount you move can reduce inflammation and its related symptoms.

→ Movement of all kinds can also help reduce or manage stress, which in turn reduces inflammation.

→ Even though some kinds of movement (like intense exercise) can increase the body's stress response in the short term, it's a healthy kind of stress. In fact, it helps turn off overactive stress and inflammatory responses.

→ Small shifts in your everyday life, like moving enough to make it a little harder to talk and incorporating three sessions of movement into your week, can make big differences in your mental health and your quality of life.

CHAPTER SIX

———

REST TO REPAIR THE BRAIN

As an accountant, Ash knows that January is stressful. Corporate clients suddenly send in thousands of year-end financial documents, and Ash's firm is all hands on deck. It's the same way every year.

Even so, this year feels different.

On one hand, Ash has more high-profile, big-name clients than ever before. It's exciting. Ash loves managing the big clients, pulling together thousands of financial puzzle pieces to create a picture of the whole year's losses and gains. The clients love Ash's meticulous work. Plus, the fact that Ash has been given all these new clients is a good sign for that promotion they've been pushing for.

On the other hand, Ash is struggling. Ash has had depression since their teens, and they've more or less managed it. With all these new clients and all the work stress, though, it's getting harder to keep the symptoms from impacting their work.

Despite the depression, Ash has been forcing themself to work the long days and nights that are needed, travel to meet with clients, and keep up with their increasingly demanding work. But the harder they push, the harder it is to bounce back. In their limited free time, all Ash can do is veg—watching TV, not going out with friends, not feeling able to do much of anything.

More recently, they've noticed cognitive challenges as well. They keep forgetting basic things. Their energy is way down, and everything seems to take twice as long to complete. As a result, their productivity is down—and that's just increasing their stress. This is not a good time of year, or a good moment in their career, for this to be happening.

For now, Ash is managing. Nothing has slipped at work yet. But it feels like just a matter of time.

Ash sets up an appointment with their doctor. The doctor asks Ash about their lifestyle, and Ash pours out their story of long days, overnight travel, and new client meetings.

When Ash is finished, the doctor looks solemn and says, "If you don't prioritize rest, your body will force you to do it." It turns out that the stress, the travel, and the long days have been pushing sleep lower and lower on Ash's priority list. The doctor warns that if they keep robbing their body of rest, it will keep forcing them to slow down in whatever way it can. The doctor also explains that lack of sleep can worsen depression symptoms.

Ash leaves the office a bit shaken but determined. Ash has always done what they need to do to succeed. Right now, it looks like that means finding ways to get more rest.

THE POWER OF REST

Rest can mean a lot of different things. It can mean taking it easy. Recharging. Slowing down. Regrouping. Pausing.

I define rest as an intentional stop, a period of not "doing" anything, in order to relax and regroup. That can mean five minutes of listening to *Enya's Greatest Hits* with my eyes closed in the middle of a barrage of Zoom meetings, a power nap in my car after a stressful Costco shopping trip, or simply lying down for a bit when I feel the exhaustion creeping in.

As Ash is finding out, rest is absolutely necessary for mental and physical health. Without it, nothing else can function properly.

The most critical form of rest is *sleep*.

Of all the actions you can take to reduce inflammation and improve your mental health, getting enough high-quality sleep is the most important.

Fueling your cells with nutrients is vital. Moving your body to increase your heart rate and improve blood flow is fundamental. Sleep is critical.

If you eat poorly over years or decades, your physical and mental health can suffer substantially. But like the diesel truck, you can keep running for a long time. A sedentary lifestyle is both a cause of inflammation and a risk factor for many diseases, but again, the effects can take months or years to show up.

An absence of sleep, on the other hand, is life-threatening.

Take Silvano. At 53, Silvano suddenly couldn't sleep anymore. No matter what he did, nothing worked. His mind and body simply wouldn't shift into sleep mode.

Just a few months later, Silvano was dead.

It turns out he had a rare genetic disease called fatal familial insomnia (FFI). FFI is a terrifying condition that shows up in middle age and damages part of the brain that regulates sleep. Remember when we talked about the HPA axis? The "H" part, the hypothalamus, works together with the thalamus (the central receiving station for all sensory information) to regulate heart rate, blood pressure, and body temperature, and FFI severely damages the thalamus. In FFI, it's as if the body's central heating goes haywire, and all your systems collapse. So far, FFI is always fatal.[88]

That's a pretty extreme example. But even a relatively low-level lack of sleep, such as being mildly sleep-deprived over a long period

---

88   David Robson, "The Tragic Fate of the People Who Stop Sleeping," *BBC Future*, January 19, 2016, https://www.bbc.com/future/article/20160118-the-tragic-fate-of-the-people-who-stop-sleeping.

of time, can have serious effects.[89] People who don't get enough sleep are more likely to catch the common cold.[90] They're also more likely to develop cancer or die of heart disease.[91]

After even one night of sleep deprivation, your brain becomes more emotionally reactive, pushing you into the fight-or-flight stress response.[92]

More recently, sleep deprivation has been shown to increase your likelihood of getting COVID-19. One 2020 study, for example, found that a *single extra hour of sleep* reduced participants' odds of getting COVID-19 by 12 percent.[93] Sleep impacts the immune system directly, increasing the risk of infection—and inflammation.

Sleep *matters*. And more broadly, *rest* matters.

Rest is about more than just feeling upbeat in the morning or not nodding off at your desk. It's about giving your body and brain the time they need to heal and repair.

We'll talk later in the chapter about how to improve the quality of your sleep. But when it comes to rest, the key is quantity: simply getting enough.

RESTING UP, NOT SHUTTING DOWN

When you sleep, your conscious mind goes dark. As a result, it can feel like your brain is simply switching off. Shutting down.

Nothing could be further from the truth.

---

89 E. H. During and M. Kawai, "Chapter Three—The Functions of Sleep and the Effects of Sleep Deprivation," in *Sleep and Neurologic Disease*, ed. Mitchell G. Miglis (Amsterdam: Elsevier, 2017), 55–72.

90 A. Wilder-Smith et al., "Impact of Partial Sleep Deprivation on Immune Markers," *Sleep Medicine* 14, no. 10 (October 2013): 1031–34, https://doi.org/10.1016/j.sleep.2013.07.001.

91 Rong Yuan, Jie Wang, and Li-li Guo, "The Effect of Sleep Deprivation on Coronary Heart Disease," *Chinese Medical Sciences Journal* 31, no. 4 (December 2016): 247–53, https://doi.org/10.1016/S1001-9294(17)30008-1.

92 Ellemarije Altena et al., "The Bidirectional Relation between Emotional Reactivity and Sleep: From Disruption to Recovery," *Behavioral Neuroscience* 130, no. 3 (2016): 336–50, https://psycnet.apa.org/doi/10.1037/bne0000128.

93 Hyunju Kim et al., "COVID-19 Illness in Relation to Sleep and Burnout," *BMJ Nutrition, Prevention, & Health* 4, no. 1 (2021), https://doi.org/10.1136/bmjnph-2021-000228.

The brain remains remarkably active during sleep. The reason you don't notice is that the patterns of activity change.[94]

During the day, our neurons are busy running our bodies. They're signaling. Connecting. Sending messages and coordinating the body's entire symphony of responses, from breathing and blinking to throwing a football or pulling up a spreadsheet. There's so much happening while you're awake that your brain never gets the chance to recover. It's like a production line worker. The conveyor belt keeps moving. The brain can't step away for lunch or clock out. It's always on duty.

When you sleep, the brain is finally able to catch up.[95] New information gathered during the day is organized and stored.[96] New connections are made or strengthened.[97] Damaged connections are repaired.[98] Energy is restored.[99] Waste byproducts that have accumulated throughout the day are power washed away.[100]

Sleep also helps improve memory. One 2019 study showed that students performed better on an exam if they napped between their study session and the exam itself. These students even performed better than the students who crammed for an extra hour instead of napping, *and* they retained the information better when tested again

94 Gabrielle Girardeau and Vítor Lopes-Dos-Santos, "Brain Neural Patterns and the Memory Function of Sleep," *Science* 374, no. 6567 (October 28, 2021): 560–64, https://doi.org/10.1126/science.abi8370.

95 J. Allan Hobson, "Sleep Is of the Brain, by the Brain and for the Brain," *Nature* 437 (October 2005): 1254–56, https://doi.org/10.1038/nature04283.

96 Monika Schönauer, Melanie Grätsch, and Steffen Gais, "Evidence for Two Distinct Sleep-Related Long-Term Memory Consolidation Processes," *Cortex* 63 (February 2015): 68–78, https://doi.org/10.1016/j.cortex.2014.08.005.

97 Wei Li et al., "REM Sleep Selectively Prunes and Maintains New Synapses in Development and Learning," *Nature Neuroscience* 20 (March 2017): 427–37, https://doi.org/10.1038/nn.4479.

98 Andy R. Eugene and Jolanta Masiak, "The Neuroprotective Aspects of Sleep," *MEDtube Science* 3, no. 1 (March 2015): 35–40, https://www.ncbi.nlm.nih.gov/pmc/articles/PMC4651462/.

99 Mindy Engle-Friedman, "The Effects of Sleep Loss on Capacity and Effort," *Sleep Science* 7, no. 4 (December 2014): 213–24, https://doi.org/10.1016/j.slsci.2014.11.001.

100 Lulu Xie et al., "Sleep Drives Metabolite Clearance from the Adult Brain," *Science* 342, no. 6156 (October 18, 2013): 373–77, https://doi.org/10.1126/science.1241224.

a week later. Sleeping allowed their brains to lock in their memories of the material and improved their ability to recall it.[101]

In other words, the work their brains did while they were asleep was every bit as important as the intentional studying they did while they were awake.

GOING DEEPER: THE STAGES OF SLEEP

Sleep isn't just one thing. Part of what makes sleep so restorative is that there are multiple stages, each with its own effects. And getting enough sleep is important in part because you need to complete all the stages every night (often several times each) to get the full benefit.

Stage One: Transition Sleep

The transition period is just what it sounds like. During the first few minutes after you fall asleep, your brain starts to slow down from the busyness and activity of the day. Your body also starts to settle down during this period. Often, your muscles will twitch as they work off energy.

Stage Two: Light Sleep

After the transition period, your breathing and heart rate slow down, your core temperature decreases, and your brain slows down even more. During this sleep stage, your brain begins to show consistent little bursts of activity called *spindles*. These are believed to be the beginning of memory consolidation: the process by which your brain gathers, processes, and filters new memories acquired during the day.[102]

---

101 James N. Cousins et al., "The Long-Term Memory Benefits of a Daytime Nap Compared with Cramming," *Sleep* 42, no. 1 (January 2019): zsy207, https://doi.org/10.1093/sleep/zsy207.

102 Gordon B. Feld and Susanne Diekelmann, "Sleep Smart—Optimizing Sleep for Declarative Learning and Memory," *Frontiers in Psychology* 6 (May 11, 2015), https://doi.org/10.3389/fpsyg.2015.00622.

Stage Three: Deep Sleep

This is where the big stuff happens. Deep sleep is the most restorative, allowing your body to recover from the activity of the day and repair systems that have been damaged. Deep sleep is believed to support the immune system, along with other key body systems. Plus, deep sleep is good for your mind.

Even though brain activity is lower during this period, evidence suggests that deep sleep helps you have more insights, be more creative, and develop what are called *declarative memories*.[103] Declarative memories are facts and events that you lock into long-term memory, like the look on your best friend's face when you jumped out at her surprise birthday party or the list of US state capitals you memorized for extra credit in fourth grade.

Stage Four: REM Sleep

REM stands for Rapid Eye Movement. While you're dreaming, your eyes move back and forth inside your eyelids, and your brain activity, breathing, and heart rate speed up, closer to where they are when you're awake. REM sleep is critical for emotional processing and for consolidating procedural and emotional memories.[104] Unlike declarative memory, procedural memory is like "muscle memory." If you've ever realized you still remember how to play "Hot Cross Buns" on a clarinet you haven't touched since fourth grade, or found yourself able to swing and hit a baseball without thinking because you've spent so many hours practicing—that's procedural memory.

REM is also one of the most important stages of sleep for mental

---

103 Juliana Yordanova et al., "Differential Associations of Early- and Late-Night Sleep with Functional Brain States Promoting Insight to Abstract Task Regularity," *PLoS One* 5, no. 2 (February 2010): e9442, https://doi.org/10.1371/journal.pone.0009442; Valeria Drago et al., "Cyclic Alternating Pattern in Sleep and its Relationship to Creativity," *Sleep Medicine* 12, no. 4 (April 2011): 361–66, https://doi.org/10.1016/j.sleep.2010.11.009; and Girardeau and Lopes-Dos-Santos, "Brain Neural Patterns and the Memory Function of Sleep."

104 Jan Born, "Slow-Wave Sleep and the Consolidation of Long-Term Memory," *World Journal of Biological Psychiatry* 11, supplement 1 (2010): 16–21, https://doi.org/10.3109/15622971003637637.

health. In addition to improving problem-solving and creativity (which can make us more resilient), it actually helps reduce the pain from traumatic events.[105] And not getting enough REM makes us feel worse generally and react more to negative events.[106] That's worth prioritizing a few hours of shut-eye.

YOU CAN'T CATCH UP

Even those of us who understand the value of sleep sometimes don't get enough. Usually, what we tell ourselves is that we'll "catch up." *It's okay*, we say to ourselves. *I'll just get a little extra sleep tomorrow.*

Unfortunately, it doesn't work that way.

The evidence is clear. Adults need seven to nine hours of sleep a night. *Every* night. Otherwise, problems start piling up.[107]

Every task your body and brain perform during the day requires energy. Every action, every decision—even simple motions like holding a coffee cup—all go through the brain, and every one takes a little bit of work. When you eat breakfast, the brain has to signal the release of digestive hormones. When you text your boss, your brain coordinates your language centers and motor response to turn your thoughts into words on the screen.

Every. Single. Action. All. Day. Long.

No wonder you need rest!

Missing sleep means that your brain's energy store—its ability to do normal, everyday tasks as well as tough ones like healing—is low. The more sleep you miss, the lower your reserves. It becomes like trying to fill a bucket with a hole in it. The longer you lose out on optimal sleep, the bigger the hole gets.

---

105 Matthew Walker, *Why We Sleep: Unlocking the Power of Sleep and Dreams* (New York: Scribner, 2017).

106 Robert W. Glosemeyer et al., "Selective Suppression of Rapid Eye Movement Sleep Increases Next-Day Negative Affect and Amygdala Responses to Social Exclusion," *Scientific Reports* 10 (October 14, 2020): 17325, https://doi.org/10.1038/s41598-020-74169-8.

107 Shingo Kitamura et al., "Estimating Individual Optimal Sleep Duration and Potential Sleep Debt," *Scientific Reports* 6 (October 24, 2016): 35812, http://dx.doi.org/10.1038/srep35812.

How big?

Let me put it this way. It takes *four days* to fully recover from *one hour* of lost sleep.[108]

Four. *Days.*

If you're regularly missing out on an hour or two a night, think how quickly you're going to get deep in debt. By the second week or so, you're so far behind that there aren't hours to make up the difference.

To make matters worse, being tired during the day makes everything you do just a bit more difficult. Your brain isn't ready for the day, so it has to work harder, causing you to need more rest and putting you that much more behind.

In other words, sleep deprivation is cumulative. It's not just a matter of getting a couple of extra hours on the weekend. Eventually, the bucket is just empty.

That's why long-term sleep deprivation is so damaging. Over time, sleep deprivation can impair memory, worsen focus and concentration, lower your ability to control your emotions, and increase your likelihood of experiencing mental illnesses from psychiatric conditions to Alzheimer's disease. Sleep deprivation is linked to a shorter life span and a host of diseases like cancer and heart disease. And people with insomnia are *ten times* more likely to experience depression.[109]

Sadly, there's no quick fix or replacement. Caffeine or energy drinks might make you feel more productive despite being sleep-deprived, but they are just putting off the inevitable.

---

108 Kitamura et al., "Estimating Individual Optimal Sleep Duration and Potential Sleep Debt."

109 Walker, *Why We Sleep.*

THE SIREN SONG OF CAFFEINE

Aaaah, the lure of the quick fix. I can totally relate. After a sleepless night or at the end of a hard week, when your brain feels like it just won't come online properly—caffeine calls to you. The drip of the coffee maker or the quick jolt of an energy drink can be the most appealing thing in the world. Unfortunately, while caffeine may make you temporarily more productive, it's just prolonging the problem.

You feel tired in large part because of a natural molecule called *adenosine*. When you are awake and active, your cells use energy, and adenosine is made as a byproduct. Adenosine builds up in your brain during the day, and as the level increases, it signals to the brain that you need to sleep. The more adenosine builds up, the more tired you feel.

The caffeine molecule looks a lot like an adenosine molecule. When you drink that cup of coffee, the caffeine molecule binds to the receptors that would normally bind with adenosine. Fewer adenosine molecules hook up to their receptors, and as a result, your brain is tricked into thinking you're not tired.

But the adenosine doesn't just go away. It floats around in the bloodstream, and once the caffeine wears off…the floating adenosine overwhelms the receptors, and…you *crash*.

Sometimes we can't avoid using caffeine, but whenever possible, it's better to grab a quick nap or even take a brisk walk to get your energy levels up again so you can sleep better tonight. And if you do use caffeine, keep it early in the day and as minimal as you can.

THE INFLAMMATION CONNECTION

When I was in college, I had a roommate who was a *terrible* procrastinator. Every time a paper was due, she would wait until she had only a few days left before she started working on it.

Early in the semester, she was okay. Her papers were rushed, but she worked well under pressure, so it was all right. The problem was that every time she put something off, it got added to the growing pile of stuff she was putting off. Then when she tried to tackle the work, there was too much of it. She couldn't get it all done. Some of it got pushed back further—pushing other stuff even further back. Eventually, she couldn't make any of her deadlines.

About two thirds of the way through the semester, the system broke down. The amount of work still left to do was impossible to complete in the time she had left.

Lack of rest and inflammation follow that same kind of self-reinforcing cycle.

Sleep deprivation leads to inflammation. Inflammation causes sleep problems. Sleep problems cause stress. Stress leads to inflammation, which leads to sleep problems, which causes stress.

Let's look at that in more detail.

We know that lack of rest leads to inflammation because people who are sleep-deprived show higher levels of blood markers of inflammation. One study of college soccer players showed just how quickly this can happen. The first night of the study, the players slept for a healthy seven and a half hours, and the researchers measured their baseline IL-6 levels (that's a pro-inflammatory cytokine, like we talked about in Chapter Three).

The next day, the researchers woke the players up really early in the morning, after just four hours of sleep, and asked them to cycle on a stationary bike as hard as they could for 30 seconds to stay awake. They took IL-6 measurements again, both before and after the exercise. What they found was that after *just one night* of sleep deprivation, despite being young and otherwise healthy, the athletes' inflammation levels went up—and stayed up throughout the day.[110]

Since then, many studies have linked sleep deprivation with

---

110 Salma Abedelmalek et al., "Effect of Time of Day and Partial Sleep Deprivation on Plasma Concentrations of IL-6 during a Short-Term Maximal Performance," *European Journal of Applied Physiology* 113 (June 8, 2012): 241–48, https://doi.org/10.1007/s00421-012-2432-7.

neuroinflammation-related disorders including depression, anxiety, fibromyalgia, multiple sclerosis, dementia, and Parkinson's disease.[111]

It's a problem Ash knows all too well. When they get enough sleep, they manage to keep the depression at bay, even during stressful periods. But when travel and work dig into their sleep schedule, the depression creeps back in—making it harder to sleep. Plus, once they are sleep-deprived, Ash is more likely to get sick, and that makes sleeping harder and work more stressful, and the cycle gets pushed up a notch.

INFLAMMATION IS A REAL HEADACHE

Ash has another reason to think about the role of inflammation in their life: their migraines.

Migraines are complex and often very difficult to treat. Scientists still don't know a lot about why some people get migraines or what causes them. What they do know is that migraines are much more than a headache. They can last days and cause nausea, numb skin, changes in how things taste or smell, and even temporary vision loss, in addition to the pain.

Recently, there's been some strong evidence suggesting that migraines might be tied to neuroinflammation.[112] This new science

---

111 Krzysztof Krysta et al., "Sleep and Inflammatory Markers in Different Psychiatric Disorders," *Psychiatry and Preclinical Psychiatric Studies* 124 (2017): 179–86, https://doi.org/10.1007/s00702-015-1492-3; Shaffi Manchanda et al., "Low-Grade Neuroinflammation Due to Chronic Sleep Deprivation Results in Anxiety and Learning and Memory Impairments," *Molecular and Cellular Biochemistry* 449 (March 16, 2018): 63–72, https://doi.org/10.1007/s11010-018-3343-7; Rosalba Siracusa et al., "Fibromyalgia: Pathogenesis, Mechanisms, Diagnosis and Treatment Options Update," *International Journal of Molecular Sciences* 22, no. 8 (April 9, 2021): 3891, https://doi.org/10.3390/ijms22083891; H. M. B. Lunde et al., "Clinical Assessment and Management of Sleep Disorders in Multiple Sclerosis: A Literature Review," *Acta Neurologica Scandinavica* 127, no. s196 (January 2013): 24–30, https://doi.org/10.1111/ane.12046; Michael R. Irwin and Michael V. Vitiello, "Implications of Sleep Disturbance and Inflammation for Alzheimer's Disease Dementia," *Lancet Neurology* 18, no. 3 (March 2019): 296–306, https://doi.org/10.1016/S1474-4422(18)30450-2; and Nicolaas I. Bohnen and Michele T. M. Hu, "Sleep Disturbance as Potential Risk and Progression Factor for Parkinson's Disease," *Journal of Parkinson's Disease* 9, no. 3 (July 30, 2019): 603–614, https://doi.org/10.3233/jpd-191627.

112 Rakesh Malhotra, "Understanding Migraine: Potential Role of Neurogenic Inflammation," *Annals of Indian Academy of Neurology* 19, no. 2 (April–June 2016): 175–82, https://pubmed.ncbi.nlm.nih.gov/27293326/.

might even lead to new treatments for migraines, which have been very hard to come by.[113]

The good news is that anything Ash does to reduce inflammation is likely to help with their migraines as well.

TWO-WAY STREET

It turns out that sleep itself is directly connected to your immune system.[114] You can see this connection when you catch the flu. As your immune system is activated to fight the infection, it also tells the body and brain to sleep more to conserve precious infection-battling energy. Sleep directly supports your recovery and repair functions.[115]

But connections go both ways.

An overactive immune response (like chronic inflammation) sends haywire signals to the brain about sleep. It tells the brain mixed messages: *Stay awake to keep your battalions engaged! Go to sleep to clean up the damage! Two hours is enough sleep—it's time to do battle again!*

So even as sleep issues cause inflammation, that inflammation turns around and causes sleep problems, ramping up the vicious cycle.

Like I said before, you can't exactly catch up. But fortunately, you can take action.

POWER UP YOUR REST

I almost hate to say that some sleep is better than other sleep. There's no kind of "high-quality" sleep that will make up for not getting

113 Oguzhan Kursun et al., "Migraine and Neuroinflammation: The Inflammasome Perspective," *Journal of Headache and Pain* 22 (June 10, 2021): 55, https://doi.org/10.1186/s10194-021-01271-1.

114 Michael R. Irwin, "Sleep and Inflammation: Partners in Sickness and in Health," *Nature Reviews Immunology* 19 (July 9, 2019): 702–715, https://doi.org/10.1038/s41577-019-0190-z.

115 Luciana Besedovsky, Tanja Lange, and Monika Haack, "The Sleep-Immune Crosstalk in Health and Disease," *Physiological Reviews* 99, no. 3 (July 2019): 1325–80, https://doi.org/10.1152/physrev.00010.2018.

enough. Just like you can't catch up by sleeping more tomorrow, you can't make up for less sleep by getting "better" sleep.

That said, there are things you can do to improve the quality of your sleep—or reduce it.

Improvers are behaviors or conditions that boost the quality of your sleep. The improvers that have the most impact on sleep are darkness, consistency, temperature, and tiredness.

In general, it's best to sleep during the hours of darkness (a.k.a., at night). Our bodies live according to something called a *circadian rhythm*. *Circa* is Latin for "about" or "around," and *dies* refers to "the day." So a circadian rhythm is our body's natural up-and-down response to the time of day. We tend to be more energized during some parts of the day and more tired during others. Naturally, we are most tired during the dark hours, so sleeping when it's dark matches and aligns the circadian rhythm, making it easier to sleep more deeply. For some shift workers, this isn't possible, but it's best to try to get as close as you can.

Consistency also improves sleep quality by locking in your circadian rhythm. The more elements of your sleep pattern you can keep consistent from one day to the next, the better. Going to bed at the same time, getting up around the same time, sleeping for the same number of hours, and so on (even on weekends!) can improve your sleep every night of the week.

Temperature is a critical part of maintaining your body's balance state (homeostasis) and circadian rhythm, and it fluctuates throughout the day, starting out warm and cooling off in the evening.[116] Being the right temperature can significantly affect sleep quality by influencing your body's ability to fall asleep, stay asleep, and experience restorative sleep. The Centers for Disease Control and Prevention recommends setting your bedroom thermostat to between 60 and 67 degrees Fahrenheit.

The final "improver" is being aware of how tired you really are. If

---

[116] Daniel J. West et al., "The Influence of the Time of Day on Core Temperature and Lower Body Power Output in Elite Rugby Union Sevens Players," *Journal of Strength and Conditioning Research* 28, no. 6 (June 2014): 1524–28, https://doi.org/10.1519/jsc.0000000000000301.

possible, it's best to go to sleep when you feel calm and tired but not utterly exhausted. Exhaustion is a sign that you're behind on sleep, which may actually keep your brain running while you're trying to fall asleep. Unfortunately, exhaustion and deep fatigue are common experiences for those of us with mental health issues. To improve your sleep, try taking naps during the day to reduce exhaustion or giving yourself more time to fall asleep at night.

Impactors are behaviors and conditions that negatively affect sleep quality. Caffeine, digestion, alcohol, blue light, and nighttime exercise are the most common.

Caffeine and digestion are both related to timing. Drinking your last cup of coffee in the late afternoon is going to make it very hard to sleep, and especially hard to sleep deeply enough for your brain to do its repair work. Caffeine can affect sleep for as much as eight hours, so cut yourself off early.

Digestion can also affect sleep. High fat and high carbohydrate foods, for example, have been shown to impact sleep cycles.[117] Even though it happens unconsciously, digestion takes a lot of work, and it can keep your body and brain active long after you eat. Although scientists don't yet agree on the ideal timing of dinner, finishing the last meal of your day at least a few hours before you plan to sleep is probably a safe bet.[118]

Alcohol can seem like it helps you sleep. It might make you feel drowsy, or even cause you to fall asleep more easily. But alcohol actually negatively impacts sleep quality, often causing you to wake up in the night and miss necessary sleep cycles. It also keeps your brain from properly processing and repairing during the night, making your sleep less effective.[119]

---

117 Katsuhiko Yajima et al., "Effects of Nutrient Composition of Dinner on Sleep Architecture and Energy Metabolism during Sleep," *Journal of Nutritional Science* 60, no. 2 (2014): 114–21, https://doi.org/10.3177/jnsv.60.114.

118 Daisy Duan et al., "Effects of Dinner Timing on Sleep Stage Distribution and EEG Power Spectrum in Healthy Volunteers," *Nature and Science of Sleep* 13 (May 14, 2021): 601–612, https://doi.org/10.2147/NSS.S301113.

119 Ian M. Colrain, Christian L. Nicholas, and Fiona C. Baker, "Alcohol and the Sleeping Brain," *Handbook of Clinical Neurology* 125 (2014): 415–31, https://doi.org/10.1016/B978-0-444-62619-6.00024-0.

Remember how sleep is important for learning and memory? Alcohol in particular can impair that process. Even healthy college students can't learn as well when they drink at night. One study, for example, found that drinking at bedtime impaired students' ability to perform new tasks they had just learned. It also reduced their ability to get into REM sleep, which is necessary for locking in memories.[120]

Certain kinds of light can also affect sleep. Natural morning light helps us to wake up, whereas natural evening light helps us shut down. Morning light is heavy with blue wavelengths, while evening light has more reddish wavelengths. Turns out, LED screens (like on televisions, computers, and phones) also put off a lot of blue light. So if you use them at night, these devices can trigger your "wake up, it's morning!" response and suppress your "fall asleep" response. If limiting your exposure to blue light altogether around bedtime isn't possible, consider using a blue-light-blocking filter. They've been found to improve sleep quality in students who use their screens around bedtime.[121]

Finally, although getting enough movement during the day can improve sleep, exercising too close to bedtime may make it hard to wind down. While moderate exercise may not have an effect, it's best to wrap up activities that noticeably increase your heart rate two to four hours before bedtime.[122] This gives your core plenty of time to cool down in time for sleep.

So while getting enough sleep, every day, is the key to resting and repairing, increasing your improvers and reducing your impactors

120 J. Todd Arnedt et al., "Sleep following Alcohol Intoxication in Healthy, Young Adults: Effects of Sex and Family History of Alcoholism," *Alcohol: Clinical & Experimental Research* 35, no. 5 (May 2011): 870–78, https://doi.org/10.1111/j.1530-0277.2010.01417.x.

121 S. A. R. Mortazavi et al., "Blocking Short-Wavelength Component of the Visible Light Emitted by Smartphones' Screens Improves Human Sleep Quality," *Journal of Biomedical Physics and Engineering* 8, no. 4 (December 2018): 375–80, https://doi.org/10.31661/jbpe.v8i4Dec.647.

122 D. J. Miller et al., "Moderate-Intensity Exercise Performed in the Evening Does Not Impair Sleep in Healthy Males," *European Journal of Sport Science* 20, no. 1 (February 2020): 80–89, https://doi.org/10.1080/17461391.2019.1611934; and Shiro Oda and Kazuki Shirakawa, "Sleep Onset is Disrupted following Pre-Sleep Exercise that Causes Large Physiological Excitement at Bedtime," *European Journal of Applied Physiology* 114, no. 9 (September 2014): 1789–99, https://doi.org/10.1007/s00421-014-2873-2.

can improve the quality of rest you're getting and help you get more sleep, more often, and for longer.

I DON'T REMEMBER BUYING THAT ON EBAY

Do you remember that meme a while ago called "Ambien Walrus"? The Ambien Walrus was a cartoon character who showed up and gave people bad ideas when they took Ambien™, like buying expensive items online or eating an entire box of cookies while they were asleep.

The weird thing is that some of the Ambien Walrus stories were based on real life. Sleep aid use has been associated with complex side effects like sleepwalking, sleep driving (!!), and other activities that users don't remember when they wake up. Withdrawal from these drugs can also cause rebound insomnia (worse than before you took them), panic attacks, and even seizures.[123]

Prescription sleep aids like benzodiazepines and zolpidem (i.e., Ambien) enhance the effect of the neurotransmitter GABA in the brain. GABA plays a vital role in falling asleep, reducing brain activity and promoting relaxation.[124] The danger with sleep aids that bind to GABA is that you can develop a dependence on them—or find yourself driving on the highway without knowing how you got there.

In 2019, the FDA announced that Ambien, and other prescription sleep medications, require a black box warning to alert users to the potential dangers. If you plan to use sleep aids, even melatonin or other "natural" options, always use them under the guidance of a healthcare professional.

---

123 Massimiliano Aragona, "Abuse, Dependence, and Epileptic Seizures after Zolpidem Withdrawal: Review and Case Report," *Clinical Neuropharmacology* 23, no. 5 (September 2000): 281–83, https://doi.org/10.1097/00002826-200009000-00008.

124 W. Wisden, X. Yu, and N. P. Franks, "GABA Receptors and the Pharmacology of Sleep," in *Sleep-Wake Neurobiology and Pharmacology*, ed. Hans-Peter Landolt and Derk-Jan Dijk (New York: Springer, 2019), 279–304.

AM I GETTING ENOUGH SLEEP?

It turns out that we're not always great at knowing whether we're getting enough sleep. Many of us have been so sleep-deprived for so long that it feels like a natural state.

In other words, "How sleepy do I feel?" doesn't begin to capture the reality.

Instead, use the following two questions to find out whether you are getting enough sleep.

1. Could I fall back asleep at 10:00 a.m. or 11:00 a.m.?
2. Can I function optimally without caffeine before noon?

All of us feel sleepy, or even exhausted, at night before bed. But morning should be the most wide-awake time of day. If you feel ready to go back to sleep in the late morning, or if you don't feel like you can function at your best before noon without that coffee boost, you probably need more sleep.

RECOMMENDATIONS

So what's the min/max on sleep? Where are the "small wins" you can incorporate to start reducing neuroinflammation and improving your mental health?

I can't stress enough that the most important recommendation for sleep and rest is *getting enough of it*. Sleep is the most powerful predictor of brain health.

If you can't do anything else in this book, try to go to bed 10 to 15 minutes earlier every night until you get as close to the recommended amount as possible. It's that important.

Sleep quality matters too. Every day, think about small ways you can increase your "improvers" and decrease your "impactors." Small changes like having that last cup of coffee earlier in the day or trying to get to bed around the same time every night can have huge benefits.

Starting the darkness cycle early can help too. Turn down the lights, turn off your screens, and start getting ready for bed before it's actually time to sleep. The increased darkness signals to your body and brain that it's time to slip into rest and repair mode.

Also, it's pretty clear that most of us are used to feeling sleep-deprived. So much so that we often can't tell whether we're getting enough sleep, whether we're sleeping well, or what we should do about it. Digital devices like Fitbits and Apple watches can show you insights you won't notice yourself, like how many times you wake up in the night or when you actually fall asleep. These insights can help you decide which small changes to make to have the biggest impact on your rest.

Finally, and I've saved this for last because it is such good news: naps are allowed! A nap isn't as good as continuous sleep, but it can definitely help.

Remember when you were in kindergarten and they let you take a nap in the middle of the day? There's a reason for that. A one-hour nap has been shown to increase learning retention in young children by 10 percent, and habitual nappers retain information for longer.[125] Even a short nap improves mental processing and gives the brain a chance to rest and repair. Naps have been shown to improve memory and even help students perform better on tests. So while overall quantity of sleep is most important, if you feel tired, take 20 to 30 minutes and give your brain a break.

125 Laura Kurdziel, Kasey Duclos, and Rebecca M. C. Spencer, "Sleep Spindles in Midday Naps Enhance Learning in Preschool Children," *Proceedings of the National Academy of Sciences USA* 110, no. 43 (2013): 17267–72, https://doi.org/10.1073/pnas.1306418110.

TOO MUCH OF A GOOD THING

Napping has a lot of benefits, but excessive napping can be a symptom of your brain and body struggling for resources. One study that looked at daytime napping changes in 1,400 older adults found that people tended to nap longer and more frequently as they aged, and longer and more frequent daytime naps were associated with a higher risk of Alzheimer's dementia.[126] Mental health issues such as depression are also correlated with a higher rate of daytime napping.[127]

Now you're probably thinking to yourself: This whole chapter is about getting me to sleep more, and now that's an issue *too*? I know. It's a lot. But here's the takeaway: if you're outside the "normal" range of sleep—either too little or too much—using the tools in this book can help level you out, whichever direction your brain and body need to go. And if you find yourself needing to nap *every* day, talk to your healthcare provider about why that might be happening.

MAKING SLEEP A PRIORITY

Whatever else is going on in their life, Ash has never been one to sit on their hands when there's something to be done. Right after meeting with their doctor, they ordered a new mattress, set up their Fitbit to monitor their sleep, and created a new sleep routine that gets them to bed almost an hour earlier than they were before. As hard as it was, they even cut out coffee after noon.

No more of those late night "just one more episode" Parks and Rec marathons with a glass of Merlot. Actually, Ash thought they'd

---

126 Peng Li et al., "Daytime Napping and Alzheimer's Dementia: A Potential Bidirectional Relationship," *Alzheimer's & Dementia* 19, no. 1 (January 2023): 158–68, https://doi.org/10.1002/alz.12636.

127 Yuning Liu et al., "The Relationship between Depression, Daytime Napping, Daytime Dysfunction, and Snoring in 0.5 Million Chinese Populations: Exploring the Effects of Socio-Economic Status and Age," *BMC Public Health* 18 (June 2018): 759, https://doi.org/10.1186%2Fs12889-018-5629-9.

miss that a lot more than they do. Now that they're not "winding down" until midnight, they can start their routine earlier.

Most importantly, they are now maintaining the same sleep routine on travel days and when they are out of town as they do at home. That consistency has made it easier to fall asleep and stay asleep.

At first, it didn't seem like such small changes could make a difference, but over several weeks, Ash did start to see a difference. They aren't falling into a sluggish two-hour productivity slump after lunch every day. Their memory feels like it is working right again, and their overall energy is up.

Tax day is rapidly approaching, but now, Ash thinks they can handle it.

Your body and brain have an incredible ability to repair and renew themselves. That's life-changing news for those of us with inflammation-related mental health issues. In order to perform that repair, though, we need fundamental resources.

Fuel, movement, and rest make up the foundation of your anti-inflammatory tool kit. Small, everyday tweaks to what you eat, how you move, and how much you sleep add up to big gains in mental health. Together, these small changes can start to slow the inflammation cycle, giving your brain the chance to recover.

Once you've put these changes in motion, though, what's next?

Most people with mental health issues who seek treatment are likely to be offered the dynamic duo of drugs and therapy. So that's where we'll head next, to find out what works, what to watch out for, and how to get the most out of these powerful—and extremely common—forms of treatment.

TL;DR

→ Getting enough rest (and specifically, enough sleep) is the most important thing you can do for your own mental health and to reduce the effects of inflammation in your body.

→ Sleep isn't an absence of activity. Your brain is very active during sleep—cleaning up and organizing thoughts and memories from the day, restoring brain cells, and making new connections.

→ It might feel like you can "catch up" from missed sleep by getting more later, but that's not really true, or at least it's not easy. It takes *four days* to make up for a single missed hour of sleep. It's important to prioritize getting enough sleep every day.

→ Shifts in your activities and schedule during the day, like cutting out afternoon caffeine, creating a consistent sleep routine, and avoiding blue light at night can help you get more, and better, sleep.

→ Be careful when using sleep aids and medications as they can have dangerous side effects and should be used under the supervision of a medical professional.

BRAIN BREAK

Intermission

Hey, can I just stop for a second and say how impressed I am that you are doing this work for yourself? I don't know you personally, but I do know that I've been where you are. I know exactly how hard it can be to make lifestyle changes, no matter how much they're going to benefit you.

It might help you to keep in mind that *even people with no mental health issues at all* struggle to make lasting lifestyle shifts. For those of us living with depression, anxiety, fatigue, and other mental health challenges, it can be an even bigger lift.

So I get it. I really, really do. The fact that you've gotten this far in the book, that you are taking control of your mental health and making tweaks, however small, to reduce the burden of inflammation in your life—that is impressive. Give yourself all the credit you deserve.

Making adjustments in fuel, movement, and rest can be life-changing, but the benefits can take a while to show up. Sometimes, you need help now.

That's why, for most of us, our first stop isn't lifestyle shifts but medical care.

For almost all of us, the first things we try are medication or therapy—or both. That's what our doctors recommend. It's what we see our friends and family members doing.

And there is nothing wrong with those approaches. In fact, they are often good places to start. There's a reason medication and therapy are considered the "gold standards" for most mental health issues.

But.

(You knew there'd be a but, right?)

But...not every approach, not even every "gold standard" approach, is right for everyone. Besides that, not all approaches are created equal. Some are evidence-supported and science-backed, while others are standard more because we've always done them that way than because they have clear evidence.

And then there are the other methods, the ones you might call new age or alternative. Yoga. Tai Chi. Sensory deprivation. Some of these have decades of science behind them, but where should you start?

The point is, there are a lot of options out there, and a lot of them claim to be your best option, or the gold standard, or the universal cure. In the next section, I'm going to walk you through the most commonly recommended approaches to mental health treatment, and we're going to understand, together, which ones are evidence-supported and how to choose which ones are right for you.

Before you turn the page, though, close your eyes and give yourself a moment. You've already taken in so much information, and maybe you've even adopted some new, inflammation-busting habits.

I won't lie. There's still a lot left to learn. But you've taken the first step, and that is something to celebrate.

UNPACKING THE GOLD STANDARD

From Pills to Poses

I started this book with everyday lifestyle shifts because those are actions you can take today. You can eat a little better. Get an extra hour of sleep. Move your body a bit more than you did yesterday. Taking that kind of initiative for your own mental health is super empowering, even beyond the specific benefits of the changes themselves.

Truth be told, though, that's not where I started in my own journey. I didn't learn about the inflammation-fighting power of nutrition, movement, and rest until I started doing my own research, years after my symptoms first started.

If you're reading this book, there's a good chance you started in the same place I did: the doctor's office.

When I first sought out help for my depression and anxiety and brain fog—and all the other symptoms I was experiencing—I was given two recommendations. They're the same two recommendations almost everyone with mental health challenges receives.

Medication and therapy.

Medications (like antidepressants and anti-anxiety drugs) and therapy are the most common approaches to treating mental health issues. And they can work. They can provide relief faster than lifestyle adjustments, and many of them actually reduce inflammation as well. Similarly, other commonly recommended treatments like supplements and alternative practices can help you get better, faster.

That's great news. But these interventions work because they are powerful. And their power also increases their potential for harm.

IF IT'S POWERFUL ENOUGH TO HELP, IT'S POWERFUL ENOUGH TO HURT

You're going to hear this phrase a lot, so now is a good time to get familiar with it. This book is about healing your brain. That's powerful stuff. Some of the methods I'm going to talk about have the potential to physically alter brain function or affect individual brain cells.

They have incredible potential to help. But improving your brain's health is something you want to get right. If possible, I want to help you avoid trial-and-error setbacks along the way.

Any substance, practice, or technology that is powerful enough to help heal your brain is also powerful enough to hurt.

Think about scalpels. You can't do surgery without them, but you wouldn't want a random person using one on you. A doctor with a needle can sew up a wound, but I bet you wouldn't try to do it on your own. I know I wouldn't.

The methods and practices I'm going to talk about in this section, including pharmaceuticals, supplements, therapy, and complementary medical practices, are like surgical tools. In the right hands, they have the power to heal. Used incorrectly, or for the wrong reason, they can be as dangerous as a scalpel in an untrained hand.

RIGHT DOESN'T ALWAYS MEAN "RIGHT FOR YOU"

One of the main ways these methods end up causing problems is that it is easy to find out about them and easy to access them, even if you don't know much about them.

You yourself probably have friends, coworkers, or relatives who are eager to share their experiences with whatever has helped them. When I got my first concussion, I got more suggestions than I could possibly deal with. All of these people were well meaning. They all wanted to help. And they probably all really did get some benefit from whatever they were recommending.

But I'm not them. My issues aren't their issues. My body isn't their body.

The same is true for you. Your body is unique. Your situation is not exactly like anyone else's.

Even the most well-studied, evidence-based treatments and therapies aren't right for everyone. What works for one person might not work for another, or might even be dangerous. That's especially true for the approaches in this section.

Plus, let's be real. Not every treatment you hear about from your friends or see on social media is well studied or evidence-based. Or they might be studied for a condition that's not the one you have. Or the side effects or interactions with other medications might not be well understood.

I know that for some of you, this is going to be hard. So I'm going to give you permission. Put your focus on *you*. Your genetics, your medical history, and your specific situation all influence what will work for you. It's your right to figure out the best approaches for your own symptoms and needs.

CHANNEL YOUR INNER TONY STARK

Okay, so this is about to get nerdy.

If you've ever seen the *Avengers* movies, you know that Tony Stark is a multibillionaire genius who built himself a high-tech exoskeleton, became Iron Man, and (spoiler alert) saved the world from aliens. You may also know that he doesn't like to be handed things.

Whenever someone tries to hand something to Tony Stark, he puts his hands in his pockets or leans away and says, "I don't like to be handed things." It's a funny little quirk, but it can also be a good lesson for those of us who have always politely accepted whatever we've been given.

Your mental health is a fundamental part of your quality of life. You decide what approaches are best for you. Channeling your inner Tony Stark in this case means doing your research. Don't just let a doctor or a therapist or a friend "hand you" their preferred solution. Learn about the evidence for what you're being offered, the side effects, and the possible downsides before you accept anything.

This section is the first step in that process.

———

CHAPTER SEVEN

PILLS, POTIONS, AND POWDERS

Pharmaceuticals and Supplements
Can Help or Hurt

Changing lifestyle habits to get more sleep was transformative for Ash. Tax season is feeling more manageable. But there's something on the horizon, gathering like a storm cloud. Ash recognizes it.

Despite all their positive work, the depression is coming back.

Ash has been through these cycles before. The depression has been part of their life since they first felt its dark pull just before their thirteenth birthday. They had always been really close to their family but as a young teenager they found themselves sitting up in their room, hearing the echoes of laughter coming from downstairs but feeling disconnected from it and alone. They cycled through feelings of confusion, loneliness, frustration, and anger throughout high school. And to top it off, Ash started getting migraines that sometimes lasted days.

Though school sometimes felt exhausting, Ash's only solace was in math class, where they found their natural skills at problem solving and number puzzles to be a welcome respite from the challenges and difficult feelings that seemed to follow them everywhere.

When they went off to college, the diverse and open-minded environment enabled Ash to understand their gender identity more clearly. Still struggling with depression, and processing this information, Ash turned to a supportive new friend who recommended they talk to the school psychiatrist.

He prescribed antidepressants—something called an SSRI—and recommended therapy. Ash picked up their prescription on the way home and booked their first appointment with a local therapist. Ash hoped that maybe the ordeal would finally be over.

And the drug did push the darkness back a bit. Ash was able to finish the semester. The problem was the side effects. After just a few months on the drug, Ash had gained 20 pounds. Normally a very driven person, now Ash felt lethargic. Bored. Unable to get motivated. It was like hearing the world through a pane of glass, or from deep underwater. Everything went on as normal, but Ash had lost connection to it.

The dark feelings were gone, but so were a lot of the good ones. There was no warmth and little joy. It was like the medication turned off all of Ash's emotions. They weren't sure it was worth it. And with the pressure of a full course load of accounting classes and homework deadlines every week, Ash felt like keeping up their therapy sessions was too difficult.

Eventually, they also stopped taking the SSRI. The depression came back, but in between depressed periods, Ash felt motivated again. With support from their family and college friends, they found the drive to push on and landed top of their class when they finished college.

Over the 15 years since then, Ash has been on antidepressants a number of times, and gone off them just as often. Every time the depression gets bad enough, Ash goes to their doctor to get more meds. Then, as soon as the depression lifts and the side effects get worse, Ash stops taking them.

It's a roller coaster. Down into the depression. Flattened out and lifeless on the meds. Up again briefly after stopping, feeling good and accomplishing things until the depression hits again.

This time, though, the stakes are higher than they've ever been. Ash wants that promotion. They have spent the last ten years at this company earning it.

Ash feels stuck. If the depression gets any worse, their work will suffer. They might even have to stop traveling. But if they go back to medication, they will gain all the weight back, and their motivation for work will plummet. It's hard to know which is worse. Or what other option there might be.

Unfortunately, Ash's situation is extremely common. The list of common side effects from antidepressants is, well, depressing. Emotional numbness. Reduced positive feelings. Caring less about others. Sexual difficulties. Weight gain. Even suicidal thoughts.[128]

The cure doesn't sound a lot better than the disease. For that matter, it doesn't sound all that *different*.

The reality, though, is that most people who seek help for depression are prescribed some form of medication. Along with therapy, medication is the most common treatment for a huge number of mental health problems, including not just depression but anxiety, panic disorder, and PTSD.

All too often, medication is prescribed without blood testing, despite research showing that inflammation can be tested for and is a predictor of medication efficacy.[129] (We'll get back to the inflammation connection later in the chapter.)

Before you try any drugs or supplements, it's critical for you to know what you're taking, why you're taking it, and for how long. These powerful tools can stabilize and support your mental health recovery if they're used carefully. But they can also cause serious harm.

---

128 Claire Cartwright et al., "Long-Term Antidepressant Use: Patient Perspectives of Benefits and Adverse Effects," *Patient Preference and Adherence* 10 (July 28, 2016): 1401–407, https://doi.org/10.2147/PPA. S110632.

129 Kenji Hashimoto, "Inflammatory Biomarkers as Differential Predictors of Antidepressant Response," *International Journal of Molecular Sciences* 16, no. 4 (2015): 7796–801, https://doi.org/10.3390/ ijms16047796.

Medications and supplements come in all different forms, including pills, powders, drops, gummies, injections, and lotions. You can find some of them in the discount bin at your local store, and some you can only get with a tightly controlled prescription. There are so many options, in so many different forms, making so many claims, that it can be hard to know where to start.

NOT ALL PILLS ARE CREATED EQUAL

We're going to talk about pharmaceuticals and supplements together in this chapter because they have a lot in common.

At a basic level, pharmaceuticals and supplements are substances that are ingested or injected that can change your biochemistry. In other words, what they have in common is their effect on you. Both pharmaceuticals and supplements work by changing something, often at the cellular level, inside your body. That's true even when the supplement is a concentrated version of something common or natural, like an herb.

Despite this basic similarity, though, pharmaceuticals and supplements are not the same. They're tested differently, regulated differently, and sold differently. Because they can affect your body so powerfully, it's important to understand the differences before you try any of them.

Pharmaceuticals are also called drugs or medications. What makes pharmaceuticals special is how they are regulated by the government. In the United States, for example, pharmaceutical drugs have to go through an approval process overseen by the Food and Drug Administration (FDA).

Any new drug has to be tested in something called a clinical trial. A clinical trial is a study that looks at how safe the new drug is and whether it actually works. The researcher or company that developed the drug has to prove that it does what they say it does, and does it safely. Then the FDA reviews the clinical trial data and decides whether the benefits of the new drug outweigh the risks. Other countries have similar processes for reviewing new drugs to make sure they're safe and effective.

Pharmaceutical drugs are often prescribed by a doctor, but they don't have to be. Some are sold as over-the-counter (OTC) medications, like cough syrup or Tylenol™. But whether they're prescription or OTC, no pharmaceutical drug can be sold in the United States without FDA approval.

Supplements don't have to follow the same requirements.

Supplements are substances that are intended to add to, or supplement, the nutrition you're getting from food.[130] At least, that was their original purpose. That's why they're called supplements.

Because packaged foods sometimes have less nutrition than fresh foods, some food companies add supplements directly to their products. Take a look at your cereal box, for example, and you're likely to see a list of added vitamins and minerals. Those are supplements.

You can also buy supplements separately from food. If you've been down the supplements aisle in your local drugstore, you've probably seen what a huge range of options there are. You can get everything from vitamin C to iron to echinacea. Some companies sell combinations of supplements that are supposed to help you get over jet lag or sleep better at night.

Over time, the definition of supplements, and the number and variety of supplements available, has grown a lot. The offerings now go way beyond vitamins and minerals that you might not be getting from your food. They include everything from amino acids to unpronounceable compounds like astaxanthin. The way supplements are created today is more advanced than simply extracting or isolating a compound from food or herbs; research labs are also synthesizing compounds that have specific effects on the body and the brain but have no specific source in nature.

The thing to remember is that supplements, whatever type they

---

130 US Food & Drug Administration, "FDA 101: Dietary Supplements," Consumer Updates, June 2, 2022, https://www.fda.gov/consumers/consumer-updates/fda-101-dietary-supplements.

are, don't require FDA review. Supplements are sometimes reviewed by the FDA, but only retroactively. If a lot of people get sick taking a supplement, the FDA will look into it. But the supplement doesn't have to be studied ahead of time. No clinical trials. No side effects testing. No guarantees of quality or consistency. That means literally millions of people can take a supplement, and a lot of them can be harmed by it, before its claims are verified.

That's concerning because the gray area between supplements and pharmaceuticals has recently gotten a lot grayer.

Officially, only pharmaceuticals can claim to treat or cure disease. Supplements aren't allowed to make those claims because they haven't been checked out by the FDA. But supplement ads skirt as close to the line as they can get. They don't claim to treat disease, but many claim to have positive effects on sleep, to reduce anxiety or depression, or to improve overall mental health.

There are also a lot more types of supplements on the market than there used to be, claiming to be useful for a lot more types of problems. Of extra concern is the sheer number of new supplements entering the market. While the FDA approves an average of 34 drugs per year, more than *one thousand* new supplements go on sale annually.

Plus, the ways that drugs and supplements are delivered can look very similar. Both can come in the form of pills, tinctures, powders, gummies, or even in an IV.

As if that weren't complicated enough, some of the same substances are treated differently in different parts of the world. A popular compound called *SAM-e* is available without a prescription as a supplement in the US, but it's a regulated pharmaceutical used to treat depression in Europe. Recent studies have shown that SAM-e can react negatively with other antidepressant drugs. Yet in the US, people with depression can take it without knowing the danger because it's labeled as a supplement—which means no pharmacist has a chance to check for interactions with the prescription drugs someone is taking.

So what is SAM-e? A drug or a supplement? Which should it be? The line isn't clear.

What is clear is this: just because something is marketed to you doesn't mean it's safe.

All pharmaceuticals and supplements are powerful, chemically active substances that can change and alter your bodily processes at a deep, even cellular, level. It's worth taking the time to know what you're taking, and why, before you put anything in your body.

Any pharmaceutical drug or supplement can help or harm, and a single substance can help some people and harm others.

Even the most studied, common compounds can be dangerous for *you* if you are taking other medications or have other conditions. Others may have the potential to be allies in your anti-inflammation journey. Either way, it pays to pay attention.

IT'S ALL CHEMICAL IMBALANCES—OR IS IT?

In the 1980s and 1990s, a new theory of mental health was starting to find legs. This theory has been called the *neurotransmitter theory*, or more often, the *chemical imbalance theory of mental health*.

Chances are, you've heard about this theory already. It says that mental health issues are caused by imbalances in the chemicals in your brain. These chemicals, called neurotransmitters, are messengers or connectors between neurons. They allow your brain to send and receive messages. That much is definitely true.

The theory stated that having too much or too little of these neurotransmitters *caused* all kinds of mental health issues from depression and anxiety to schizophrenia. Not exactly.

The chemical imbalance model was big news because it promised something totally new. For the first time, it was possible to create targeted drugs for mental health. Just add or subtract or rearrange the neurotransmitters in your brain, and voilà! Depression cured. Anxiety managed. Schizophrenia under control.

One neurotransmitter in particular was supposed to be responsible for a whole host of problems. That was serotonin. The idea was that the brain wasn't producing enough serotonin. Or perhaps the neurons were taking serotonin back too quickly after releasing it. Either way, serotonin was going to revolutionize depression treatment.[131]

Serotonin was the mental health breakthrough of the century. Until it wasn't.

Unfortunately, it wasn't that simple. Right off the bat, the drugs caused terrible side effects for at least some people. And even at the beginning, the new medicines worked for some people but didn't help everyone—often not even a majority of the patients they were prescribed to.

So researchers kept working on the problem. New drugs were tested. New approaches to neurotransmitter management were studied. It seemed that surely, the ideal antidepressant pill was almost within reach.

Over time, some side effects were reduced, but even the newer antidepressants retained a challenging list of side effects—some of which persisted even after patients stopped taking them.[132]

A number of very commonly prescribed antidepressants have been developed based on the neurotransmitter theory of mental health. If you are prescribed a medication for your depression, anxiety, or related symptoms, it's likely to be one of these.

If you're prescribed one of these drugs, you should know exactly what you're getting.

131 Francisco Lopez-Munoz and Cecilio Alamo, "Monoaminergic Neurotransmission: The History of the Discovery of Antidepressants from 1950s Until Today," *Current Pharmaceutical Design* 15, no. 14 (2009): 1563–86, http://dx.doi.org/10.2174/138161209788168001.

132 Michael P. Hengartner et al., "Protracted Withdrawal Syndrome after Stopping Antidepressants: A Descriptive Quantitative Analysis of Consumer Narratives from a Large Internet Forum," *Therapeutic Advances in Psychopharmacology* 10 (2020), https://doi.org/10.1177/2045125320980573.

SSRIs: THE MOST COMMON PRESCRIPTION FOR DEPRESSION

Selective serotonin reuptake inhibitors (SSRIs) are one of the most common types of drugs prescribed for mental health issues—and the most commonly prescribed for depression.[133] SSRIs are designed to increase the levels of serotonin in your brain.[134]

Let's break down "selective serotonin reuptake inhibitors" for a second.

Remember, we already talked about serotonin. It's called your *mood regulator*: it helps you stay in a good mood, if you have enough. If you don't, you can get depressed or feel down.

Reuptake is kind of a weird word, but it just means that after serotonin is released, it has to be gathered back up by your neurons. It's like recycling: your brain uses the serotonin by releasing it, then scoops it back into the neurons to use again.

An *inhibitor* is anything that slows something down or stops it from happening.

So what's an SSRI? It's a special kind of drug that keeps serotonin from going back into the neurons after it's been released. And it's "selective" because it affects only serotonin, not any of the other neurotransmitters.

The idea behind SSRIs is that, supposedly, if you keep the serotonin floating around between the neurons instead of being taken back up again, it will keep your mood high for longer. That should reduce your feelings of depression and anxiety.

But like I mentioned before, we've recently learned that this understanding of the cause of depression, and the way these drugs treat mental health issues, doesn't really capture the full story.

One especially important "umbrella" review (which looked at more than 1,000 already-published studies) found that even though

---

133 *MedlinePlus Magazine*, "Commonly Prescribed Antidepressants and How They Work," National Institute of Mental Health, September 21, 2023, https://magazine.medlineplus.gov/article/commonly-prescribed-antidepressants-and-how-they-work.

134 Andrew Chu and Roopma Wadhwa, *Selective Serotonin Reuptake Inhibitors* (Treasure Island, FL: StatPearls Publishing, 2023), https://pubmed.ncbi.nlm.nih.gov/32119293/.

the serotonin theory about depression was still influencing drug development, *there was no clear evidence that depression was caused by serotonin deficiency.*[135]

Stop and think about that for a minute. Researchers have thought for *decades* that science had already explained how these drugs work, and now they're finding out that the data says the foundation of their entire theory is *wrong.* The new findings are upending many things that were "known" about serotonin and shedding light on better, more accurate explanations of what's happening in depression.

The chemical imbalance theory was at best partially true. For many mental health issues, it was just plain wrong.

But here's where it gets even more complicated—and interesting.

If serotonin imbalance wasn't causing depression, why were the drugs working for anyone?

It turns out that SSRI drugs have an interesting side effect: they affect something other than serotonin. Something that *is* directly related to mental health.

Neuroinflammation.

What?

Yep—the newest research is showing that, despite originally being designed based on the neurotransmitter theory, SSRIs are in fact reducing inflammation. That might even be why they work to treat depression and anxiety for some people.[136]

However, even with the recent evidence that serotonin levels may not be the primary cause of mental health issues as they were thought to be, SSRIs are still very commonly prescribed for depression, anxiety, and other conditions. Because SSRIs have been linked with very severe side effects, it makes sense to ask your doctor exactly why

135 Joanna Moncrieff et al., "The Serotonin Theory of Depression: A Systematic Umbrella Review of the Evidence," *Molecular Psychiatry* 28 (July 20, 2022): 3243–56, http://dx.doi.org/10.1038/s41380-022-01661-0.

136 Vlad Dionisie et al., "The Anti-inflammatory Role of SSRI and SNRI in the Treatment of Depression: A Review of Human and Rodent Research Studies," *Inflammopharmacology* 29 (2021): 75–90, https://doi.org/10.1007/s10787-020-00777-5.

they're being prescribed for you, how long you're going to be on them, and the plan for eventually getting you off them.

OTHER COMMON MEDICATIONS

SSRIs are by far the most commonly prescribed medications for depression and anxiety, as well as some other related mental health issues. But there are some other relatively common ones we should talk about briefly.

Many of these other drugs are described by which neurotransmitters they inhibit or act on. Serotonin and norepinephrine reuptake inhibitors (SNRIs), for example, are similar to SSRIs but inhibit more than one neurotransmitter. They act on both serotonin and another chemical called *norepinephrine*. Noradrenaline and specific serotonergic antidepressants (NaSSAs) act on slightly different, more specific neurotransmitters, and some people have fewer side effects on these types of drugs.

The Tricyclic antidepressants and tetracyclic antidepressants (TCAs) are slightly different. They are called *cyclic antidepressants* for short, and they were developed before SSRIs. TCAs can help some people who don't do well on SSRIs, but they tend to have more side effects, and they have largely been replaced by SSRIs.

The most important thing to remember about SSRIs and other drugs for mental health is that none of them is a permanent fix.

Medication can be a very important bridge for some people. Getting on medication can reduce your symptoms long enough to make more lasting changes. Or you might be on medication until you can access some of the more powerful, cutting-edge approaches we'll talk about later in the book.

Help in Your Medicine Cabinet?

When I'm in pain, or I have a headache, or something just isn't feeling right, I'm always tempted to just reach in my cabinet and grab an aspirin. And strangely enough, whenever I take one, I kind of...feel better emotionally too.

Aspirin, along with ibuprofen, acetaminophen (Tylenol™), and naproxen (Aleve™), is an NSAID. That stands for *non-steroidal anti-inflammatory drug*. So here we are talking about inflammation, and we've all got anti-inflammatory drugs right in our homes already.

So I started looking into it. Could what's in your medicine cabinet already be a cheap, easy solution to your mental health issues?

The answer is: kind of, but with a big "but" attached.

One study, for example, looked at the effects of adding NSAIDs to a standard antidepressant treatment. Lo and behold, it worked. The researchers gave 40 patients with major depressive disorder the same SSRI medication, but half also got an NSAID, while the other half got a placebo. The results showed that the patients who took the NSAID had fewer depression symptoms than those who took the placebo.[137]

In fact, 95 percent of the patients who took the NSAID responded to the treatment, compared to 50 percent of those who got the placebo. And 35 percent of the people who got the NSAID had complete relief of symptoms, compared to just 5 percent in the placebo group.

But beware! NSAIDs are responsible for 30 percent of hospital admissions for adverse drug reactions, mainly due to bleeding, heart attack, and stroke.[138] Long-term use of NSAIDs is risky, so, as always, it's important to talk to a healthcare provider before taking any drug or supplement...even something as simple as aspirin.

If medication can "power down" the stress cycle long enough to start the healing process, it can be a useful part of your mental health toolbox. Just be aware of the potential side effects, the difficulties

137 Seyed-Hesameddin Abbasi et al., "Effect of Celecoxib Add-On Treatment on Symptoms and Serum IL-6 Concentrations in Patients with Major Depressive Disorder: Randomized Double-Blind Placebo-Controlled Study," *Journal of Affective Disorders* 141, no. 2–3 (December 2012): 308–314, https://doi.org/10.1016/j.jad.2012.03.033.

138 Abigail Davis and John Robson, "The Dangers of NSAIDs: Look Both Ways," *British Journal of General Practice* 66, 645 (2016): 172–73, https://doi.org/10.3399%2Fbjgp16X684433.

you might face in getting off the drug, and how long you plan to use medication while you pursue more long-term options.

SUPPLEMENTAL SUPPORT

Like medications, supplements are often recommended for mental health support but can help or harm, depending on how they're used.

Over the past couple of decades, supplements have exploded. Three out of every four adults in the US take a supplement regularly. The FDA estimates that close to 30,000 supplement products are available in the US.

That's a lot to keep track of.

Supplements range from plant products like ground-up seeds to jumbo containers of protein powder to gummy multivitamins and dropper bottles of chlorophyll.

The most common and well-known supplements tend to be things you've heard of: vitamins like vitamin C and folate, minerals like iron, or herbs like turmeric. But whole new categories of supplements are popping up all the time. In addition to the more traditional supplements, you can now buy amino acids, rare herbs, and live microbes (called probiotics). You can even buy collagen, a protein that makes up bones and muscles.

NOOTROPICS: NOT REALLY THAT NEW

You might also have heard of a popular new group of supplements called *nootropics*. A lot of claims are being made about these "brain enhancers" or "smart drugs." But don't buy the hype. *Any* drug or supplement that has a specific effect on brain function is technically nootropic. ADHD medications, caffeine, and lion's mane mushrooms are all nootropics. So are Ambien and a lot of readily available supplements.

Almost everything that affects the body also affects the mind. "Nootropic" may be an effective marketing term, but it doesn't tell you which supplements might actually be good for your mental health.

Unlike pharmaceuticals, you don't need a prescription to buy supplements. You can toss them in your cart at the supermarket or even have them delivered.

That can be great news for accessibility. It can also be a hazard.

SUPPLEMENTS GONE WRONG

While they can't legally claim to cure any disease, that doesn't stop supplement marketers from *suggesting* that their products help with issues ranging from depression and anxiety to chronic pain and even the common cold.

That can be confusing for those of us trying to figure out what will help us feel better. Remember, supplements aren't reviewed or approved by the FDA, the way drugs are. They don't go through any mandatory clinical study process. They only need to steer clear of the FDA's oversight by minimizing negative reactions and passing an occasional random audit for the purity of their product.

More to the point, even a generally safe substance might not be safe for *you*. Just ask anyone with a peanut allergy.

Supplements can be a powerful support for your mental health. They can also be a roll of the dice. And different supplements, even though they are under the same basic category, can have very different effects.

This darker side of supplements is no joke. Every year, an estimated 23,000 people end up in the emergency room because of bad reactions to supplements.[139]

---

139 Andrew I. Geller et al., "Emergency Department Visits for Adverse Events Related to Dietary Supplements," *New England Journal of Medicine* 373 (October 15, 2015): 1531–40, https://doi.org/10.1056/nejmsa1504267.

It can be very tempting to take supplements because they are easy to get and claim to have a lot of benefits. In supplements, though, like in anything else, what seems too good to be true often is.

DEADLY COMBINATIONS

Supplements are like power tools. Used for the right purpose, by a skilled craftsman, with the right safety precautions, power tools help us get the results we want with less work. In the wrong hands, without the right safety gear in place, or used for the wrong task, the same tools can be deadly.

Even well-known, widely used supplements can have dangerous side effects, especially when combined with pharmaceuticals or other supplements.

Let's look at a few examples that you might see online or at your local drugstore.

5-HTP is the chemical name for 5-hydroxytryptophan. It's related to tryptophan, a chemical your body makes when you eat certain foods like turkey. Tryptophan normally makes you feel tired. Recently, there have been a lot of claims about 5-HTP as a supplement. It's especially been marketed for depression. People who are on prescription antidepressants, who don't feel like their medications are working very well, sometimes try 5-HTP to "boost" their meds.

So what's wrong with that?

What's wrong is that when 5-HTP is combined with antidepressants, it can lead to serotonin syndrome, a terrifying overload of serotonin in the brain that can cause high fever, tremors, muscle rigidity, rapid heart rate, confusion, high blood pressure, and even death.[140] And it's not just antidepressants. 5-HTP can cause serotonin syndrome when it's combined with some migraine medications, drugs

---

140 Massimo E. Maffei, "5-Hydroxytryptophan (5-HTP): Natural Occurrence, Analysis, Biosynthesis, Biotechnology, Physiology and Toxicology," *International Journal of Molecular Sciences* 22, no. 1 (2021): 181, https://doi.org/10.3390/ijms22010181.

like Robitussin and tramadol, and likely others that haven't been identified yet.[141]

5-HTP is safe on its own; that's why it is for sale. But in certain combinations, it can be deadly. And even worse, the very people most likely to try 5-HTP—people with depression—are also the most likely to experience severe side effects.

St. John's wort is slightly better known, but in some ways it's more dangerous because it's marketed as "all natural." St. John's wort gets recommended for depression, but in addition to its other effects, it also increases the metabolism of other drugs.[142] That means that St. John's wort speeds up how fast other drugs move through your body—including antidepressants.

Most modern antidepressants are designed to be time-released. They stay in the body for a certain period of time and keep your depression symptoms at bay over that whole time. If the drug is cleared out of your body too quickly, you don't absorb it all, and you can't get the benefit. Ironically, St. John's wort may be reducing the effectiveness of antidepressants, not boosting it.[143]

There's a sense that anything that comes from a plant must be safe. Natural doesn't mean safe, though. Arsenic is natural. So is poison ivy.

Obviously, St. John's wort isn't a poison like arsenic. But like 5-HTP, it can become a problem when mixed with the wrong companions.[144]

SAM-e, like 5-HTP, can interact badly with other commonly

141 Mount Sinai, "5-Hydroxytryptophan (5-HTP)," Icahn School of Medicine at Mount Sinai, accessed March 11, 2023, https://www.mountsinai.org/health-library/supplement/5-hydroxytryptophan-5-htp.

142 Linda B. Moore et al., "St. John's Wort Induces Hepatic Drug Metabolism through Activation of the Pregnane X Receptor," *Proceedings of the National Academy of Sciences USA* 97, no. 13 (June 13, 2000): 7500–502, https://doi.org/10.1073/pnas.130155097.

143 National Center for Complementary and Integrative Health, "St. John's Wort and Depression: In Depth," National Institutes of Health, last modified November 2017, https://www.nccih.nih.gov/health/st-johns-wort-and-depression-in-depth.

144 Medsafe: New Zealand Medicines and Medical Devices Safety Authority, "Interactions with St. John's Wort (Hypericum perforatum) Preparations," Ministry of Health New Zealand, April 2000, https://www.medsafe.govt.nz/profs/puarticles/sjw.htm.

prescribed drugs and cause serotonin syndrome.[145] And although it can help people with depression, it can be dangerous for those with bipolar disorder, increasing the risk of mania.[146] In Europe, where SAM-e is only available by prescription, this risk can be monitored and carefully managed. In the US and other countries where you can buy SAM-e without a pharmacist's or doctor's oversight, it can be highly dangerous.

One last example: **kava.** Kava is made from a plant that's traditional in the South Pacific. But kava supplements are far more concentrated than the traditional form. Taken at high doses, kava can lead to hepatitis, cirrhosis, liver failure, and even death.[147] Some people have had to get liver transplants after taking too much.

Kava isn't alone in this. A lot of supplements are otherwise safe and natural substances that have been taken out of their traditional contexts, super-concentrated, bottled, and sold as if they were as safe as the original. You can't just assume that's true.

The same supplement can be effective, not effective, dangerous, or even deadly, depending on how it's taken, how concentrated it is, what it's combined with, and what form it's in.

The really scary news? This list isn't anywhere near complete.

I've only included a few of the most common, popular supplements with known side effects. *Anything* you choose to put in your body, especially in high doses, deserves a careful review.

Just because it's for sale doesn't mean it's safe.

145 L. M. Iruela et al., "Toxic Interaction of S-Adenosylmethionine and Clomipramine," *American Journal of Psychiatry* 150, no. 3 (1993): 522, https://doi.org/10.1176/ajp.150.3.522b.

146 Teodoro Bottiglieri, Patricia L. Gerbarg, and Richard P. Brown, "S-Adenosylmethionine," in *Complementary and Integrative Treatments in Psychiatric Practice*, ed. Patricia L. Gerbarg, Philip R. Muskin, and Richard P. Brown (Arlington, VA: American Psychiatric Association Publishing, 2017).

147 Peter P. Fu et al., "Toxicity of Kava Kava," *Journal of Environmental Science and Health, Part C* 26, no. 1 (2008): 89–112, https://doi.org/10.1080/10590500801907407.

CONCENTRATED INFLAMMATION FIGHTERS

When it comes to fighting inflammation, some of the most powerful supplements are also some of the simplest.

As I talked about in Chapter Four, there are certain foods that fight inflammation and reduce the impacts of the stress cycle on the body and the brain. But it can be hard to get these foods in high enough concentrations to get the benefits. Supplement versions of these foods can help you fight inflammation without having to change your entire diet.

Although most whole-plant foods provide some anti-inflammatory benefits, there are a few that are so well studied and so powerful at fighting inflammation that almost anyone could benefit from taking them.

A WALK THROUGH THE SPICE AISLE

I've always loved spices. The smell that fills the kitchen when I chop garlic or the subtle flavors of a good curry simmering in the slow cooker. So imagine my excitement when I found out that these seemingly simple ingredients were also fighting the battle against inflammation in my body!

Let's take a look at a few that have been studied extensively.

If you've ever had curry, you've definitely eaten **turmeric**. Turmeric is ground from a root and has a bright-orange color. It's been used medicinally for thousands of years, but recent research is also validating its effects.

The active ingredient in turmeric is a compound called *curcumin*. Curcumin has been shown to improve memory and mood in people with age-related memory loss and reduce the brain inflammation related to Alzheimer's and depression.[148] In one study, curcumin

---

[148] Gary W. Small et al., "Memory and Brain Amyloid and Tau Effects of a Bioavailable Form of Curcumin in Non-Demented Adults: A Double-Blind, Placebo-Controlled 18 Month Trial," *American Journal of Geriatric Psychiatry* 26, no. 3 (March 2018): 266–77, https://doi.org/10.1016/j.jagp.2017.10.010.

improved mental health, reduced inflammation, *and* lowered body weight in otherwise healthy overweight participants.[149] And a recent review of studies suggests that curcumin can be a tool in managing inflammatory conditions, metabolic syndrome, arthritis, and anxiety, among others.[150]

Ginger calls to mind the spicy fragrance of Thai food or the crisp snap of a cookie, but it's got a lot more going for it than its spicy-sweet flavor.

Many large-scale research studies have found evidence of a beneficial effect of ginger on reducing inflammation.[151] Importantly, it has been found to help with neuroinflammation specifically and may help prevent neurodegenerative diseases like Alzheimer's, Parkinson's, and multiple sclerosis, as well as neurological conditions like migraines and epilepsy.[152]

Garlic is one of my all-time favorite spices. I mean, what other food gives hummus its flavor, transforms a bland spaghetti dinner into a tempting gourmet meal—*and* deters vampires?

Kidding aside, garlic has a lot of benefits, and many of them come from a strange source: sulfur. Sulfur is the chemical that reeks in rotten eggs, and it's also the chemical that gives garlic its pungency. We don't eat a ton of sulfur because, well, in most cases it's "pungent" enough to keep away the undead. In garlic, though, not only is it delicious, but it also promotes health and prevents disease.

Garlic has been shown to be effective in managing or prevent-

149 Ryusei Uchio et al., "*Curcuma longa* Extract Improves Serum Inflammatory Markers and Mental Health in Healthy Participants Who Are Overweight: A Randomized, Double-Blind, Placebo-Controlled Trial," *Nutrition Journal* 20 (November 13, 2021): 91, https://doi.org/10.1186/s12937-021-00748-8.

150 Susan J. Hewlings and Douglas S. Kalman, "Curcumin: A Review of Its' Effects on Human Health," *Foods* 6, no. 10 (October 2017): 92, https://doi.org/10.3390/foods6100092.

151 Megan Crichton et al., "Orally Consumed Ginger and Human Health: An Umbrella Review," *American Journal of Clinical Nutrition* 115, no. 6 (June 2022): 1511–27, https://doi.org/10.1093/ajcn/nqaco35.

152 Su-Chen Ho, Ku-Shang Chang, and Chih-Cheng Lin, "Anti-Neuroinflammatory Capacity of Fresh Ginger is Attributed Mainly to 10-Gingerol," *Food Chemistry* 141, no. 3 (December 2013): 3183–91, https://doi.org/10.1016/j.foodchem.2013.06.010; and Raúl Arcusa et al., "Potential Role of Ginger (*Zingiber officinale* Roscoe) in the Prevention of Neurodegenerative Diseases," *Frontiers in Nutrition* 9 (March 18, 2022), https://doi.org/10.3389/fnut.2022.809621.

ing many common human diseases, including cancer, heart disease, high blood pressure, and diabetes.[153] Perhaps even more exciting, a variety called *black garlic* (which is aged in a way that increases its antioxidant compounds) can make your brain more resilient against neuroinflammation and neurodegeneration.[154]

I don't know about you, but in my opinion, that's worth a little garlic breath.

NATURE'S POWER HOUSES

Spices aren't the only naturally occurring inflammation busters that you can get in concentrated form. If anything, the problem is that there are too many options. I've spent plenty of time wandering down the supplement aisle wondering, *What the heck is all this stuff—and does any of it really work?*

Good news: some of it really does. Out of all the thousands of bottles on the supplement shelf, here are a few of the most beneficial.

Blueberry extract comes from, well, blueberries. Berries are packed with anti-inflammatory compounds. And blueberries in particular are high in dietary fibers and antioxidants like vitamins C, B complex, E, and A. They provide high amounts of the necessary minerals selenium, zinc, iron, and manganese, and they've got tons of other benefits, including something called *anthocyanins*, which are beneficial compounds mostly found in blue and purple foods.[155]

Small but mighty indeed.

(As an aside: I have to admit that I sometimes just love the titles of these food studies. Like "The Effect of Blueberry Interventions on

153 Johura Ansary et al., "Potential Health Benefit of Garlic Based on Human Intervention Studies: A Brief Overview," *Antioxidants* 9, no. 7 (July 15, 2020): 619, https://doi.org/10.3390/antiox9070619.

154 Tanvir Ahmed and Chin-Kun Wang, "Black Garlic and Its Bioactive Compounds on Human Health Diseases: A Review," *Molecules* 26, no. 16 (August 19, 2021): 5028, https://doi.org/10.3390/molecules26165028.

155 Katharina Miller, Walter Feucht, and Markus Schmid, "Bioactive Compounds of Strawberry and Blueberry and Their Potential Health Effects Based on Human Intervention Studies: A Brief Overview," *Nutrients* 11, no. 7 (July 2, 2019): 1510, https://doi.org/10.3390/nu11071510.

Cognitive Performance and Mood." To me, the phrase "blueberry interventions" sounds like something from *Willy Wonka and the Chocolate Factory*. Didn't somebody get turned into a blueberry in that movie? But I digress.)

Blueberry interventions are a popular area of research because blueberries have incredible anti-inflammatory potential. Blueberries, whether consumed whole or as supplements, can improve mood and even cognitive performance, especially memory.[156] A blueberry-rich diet can reduce anxiety and other signs of distress in PTSD.[157] Some of these studies are still preliminary, but even the suggestion that something as everyday as blueberries could affect PTSD is big news.

Probiotics and prebiotics are the "good" bacteria and bacteria food. As we talked about in the fuel chapter, Chapter Four, our gut contains trillions of microbiota that play a crucial role in digestion and contribute to the overall functioning of the immune system. Probiotics are "good" bacteria that we can eat to help maintain a balanced and healthy gut microbiota. Probiotics are found in certain foods like yogurt, kefir, and sauerkraut, and in dietary supplements. When you ingest probiotics, they can enhance the existing beneficial bacteria in your gut, promoting digestive health and supporting your immune system.[158]

Prebiotics are nondigestible fibers that the probiotic bacteria eat in order to grow and play their supporting role.[159] Prebiotics are like fertilizers for your gut bacteria. They are found in foods such as bananas, onions, garlic, whole grains, and certain vegetables. By

---

156 Nikolaj Travica et al., "The Effect of Blueberry Interventions on Cognitive Performance and Mood: A Systematic Review of Randomized Controlled Trials," *Brain, Behavior, and Immunity* 85 (March 2020): 96–105, https://doi.org/10.1016/j.bbi.2019.04.001.

157 Philip J. Ebenezer et al., "The Anti-Inflammatory Effects of Blueberries in an Animal Model of Post-Traumatic Stress Disorder (PTSD)," *PLoS One* 11, no. 9 (September 2016), https://doi.org/10.1371/journal.pone.0160923.

158 Marla Cunningham et al., "Shaping the Future of Probiotics and Prebiotics," *Trends in Microbiology* 29, no. 8 (August 2021): 667–85, https://doi.org/10.1016/j.tim.2021.01.003.

159 Siyong You et al., "The Promotion Mechanism of Prebiotics for Probiotics: A Review," *Frontiers in Nutrition* 9 (October 5, 2022), https://doi.org/10.3389/fnut.2022.1000517.

consuming prebiotic-rich foods, you're essentially providing nourishment for the good bacteria in your gut, helping them thrive and maintain a healthy balance.[160]

Remember that study where researchers found a clear link between gut bacteria and depression (those who were depressed had less of certain bacterias)? The researchers didn't stop at measuring those bacteria levels. They actually provided treatment to participants with depression in the form of probiotics, and the outcome was striking—participants improved in their depression symptoms just by taking probiotics regularly. That's right, nothing else changed for them, and no other treatments were done.[161]

CBD (cannabidiol) is one supplement that gets a lot more press than blueberries. There's also a lot of misinformation about it. CBD is a compound found in the cannabis plant. But that doesn't mean it will get you "high." CBD is not psychoactive, meaning it doesn't change your perception or your conscious experience of the world.

It is, however, very active against inflammation.

CBD is so effective in so many different conditions that it can be hard to believe. It can relieve both pain and spasticity (a symptom that's like constant cramping) in multiple sclerosis and reduce the nausea and vomiting that come with cancer treatments.[162] Topical CBD oil, which is rubbed onto the skin, is such an effective anti-inflammatory that some patients with arthritis can dump their painkillers altogether.[163]

CBD has been shown to reduce neuroinflammation in conditions ranging from childhood epilepsy to dementia and to be effective

---

160 You et al., "The Promotion Mechanism of Prebiotics for Probiotics."

161 Katarzyna Socała et al., "The Role of Microbiota-Gut-Brain Axis in Neuropsychiatric and Neurological Disorders," Pharmacological Research 172 (October 2021): 105840, https://doi.org/10.1016/j.phrs.2021.105840.

162 Cristina Pagano et al., "Cannabinoids: Therapeutic Use in Clinical Practice," International Journal of Molecular Sciences 23, no. 6 (March 2022): 3344, https://doi.org/10.3390/ijms23063344.

163 Pacific Rheumatology Medical Center, "CBD Oil and Inflammation: Why Some Patients Are Saying Goodbye to Ibuprofen," Pacific Rheumatology Medical Center (blog), accessed May 13, 2023, https://www.pacificrheumatologycenter.com/blog/cbd-oil-and-inflammation-why-some-patients-are-saying-goodbye-to-ibuprofen.

against both brain and intestinal inflammation in autoimmune conditions.[164] CBD reduces oxidative stress, the inflammatory stress put on cells by the "free radicals" or reactive oxygen species we talked about in Chapter Three.[165]

Bonus: CBD can control the release of pro-inflammatory chemicals in the brain, regulating neuroinflammation directly, and it shows a lot of promise in protecting against neurodegenerative disorders like Alzheimer's and Parkinson's.[166]

The extra-good news for people who have been concerned about trying other cannabis products is that CBD is generally considered safe, and there is no evidence that it causes major health problems or side effects.[167]

Last but certainly not least, **vitamin D** is a mighty little compound that plays a lot of different roles in your body. It helps you absorb minerals like calcium and magnesium, and it's involved in cell growth and maintaining the connection between the brain and the muscles, among other functions. You can get vitamin D by eating foods like fatty fish or just by getting sun on your skin.

In addition to its many other benefits, vitamin D (you guessed it) decreases biomarkers of inflammation.[168] That makes sense, since it's involved in immune function as well. Large-scale studies show

164 Brian E. Leonard and Feyza Aricioglu, "Cannabinoids and Neuroinflammation: Therapeutic Implications," *Journal of Affective Disorders Reports* 12 (April 2023): 100463, https://doi.org/10.1016/j. jadr.2023.100463; and Nicholas Dopkins et al., "Effects of Orally Administered Cannabidiol on Neuroinflammation and Intestinal Inflammation in the Attenuation of Experimental Autoimmune Encephalomyelitis," *Journal of Neuroimmune Pharmacology* 17 (November 2021): 15–32, https://doi. org/10.1007/s11481-021-10023-6.

165 Sinemyiz Atalay, Iwona Jarocka-Karpowicz, and Elzbieta Skrzydlewska, "Antioxidative and Anti-Inflammatory Properties of Cannabidiol," *Antioxidants* 9, no. 1 (2020): 21, https://doi.org/10.3390/ antiox9010021.

166 Meagan McKenna and Jason J. McDougall, "Cannabinoid Control of Neurogenic Inflammation," *British Journal of Pharmacology* 177, no. 19 (October 2020): 4386–99, https://doi.org/10.1111/bph.15208; and Sukanya Bhunia et al., "Cannabidiol for Neurodegenerative Disorders: A Comprehensive Review," *Frontiers in Pharmacology* 13 (October 24, 2022), https://doi.org/10.3389/fphar.2022.989717.

167 Kerstin Iffland and Franjo Grotenhermen, "An Update on Safety and Side Effects of Cannabidiol: A Review of Clinical Data and Relevant Animal Studies," *Cannabis and Cannabinoid Research* 2, no. 1 (June 1, 2017): 139–54, https://doi.org/10.1089/can.2016.0034.

168 K. Yin and D. Agrawal, "Vitamin D and Inflammatory Diseases," *Journal of Inflammation Research* 7 (2014): 69–87, https://doi.org/10.2147/JIR.S63898.

that low vitamin D is associated with a higher risk of depression, especially over long periods of time.[169] And older adults with higher levels of vitamin D have better cognitive function than those with lower levels, even among groups of adults who all have some age-related cognitive decline.[170]

However, a caution. Very high levels of vitamin D can cause kidney stones and other side effects, so definitely work with your doctor to find out whether your levels are low and how much, if any, you should be taking.[171]

THE OMEGA EXCEPTION

So I know I just said that everyone is different and that what works for others might not work for you. But if there's one exception to that rule, it's omega-3s.

Omega-3s are fatty acids. They are one of those "healthy fats" you've probably heard people talking about. Scientists go further. They call it an *essential* fat. That's partly because of its amazing benefits and partly because, unlike other fats, your body can't make it on its own. You *have* to get it from food.[172]

Fatty acids are incredibly important. They're the starting point for making hormones that regulate blood clotting, contraction and relaxation of your blood vessel walls, and inflammation. They also

---

169 Rebecca E. S. Anglin et al., "Vitamin D Deficiency and Depression in Adults: Systematic Review and Meta-Analysis," *British Journal of Psychiatry* 202, no. 2 (February 2013): 100–107, https://doi.org/10.1192/bjp.bp.111.106666.

170 M. Kyla Shea et al., "Brain Vitamin D Forms, Cognitive Decline, and Neuropathology in Community-Dwelling Older Adults," *Alzheimer's & Dementia* 19, no. 6 (June 2023): 2389–96, https://doi.org/10.1002/alz.12836.

171 National Institutes of Health Office of Dietary Supplements, "Vitamin D: Fact Sheet for Consumers," National Institutes of Health, last modified November 8, 2022, https://ods.od.nih.gov/factsheets/VitaminD-Consumer/.

172 Harvard T. H. Chan School of Public Health, "Omega-3 Fatty Acids: An Essential Contribution," *The Nutrition Source* (blog), accessed March 11, 2024, https://www.hsph.harvard.edu/nutritionsource/what-should-you-eat/fats-and-cholesterol/types-of-fat/omega-3-fats/.

help create and maintain the basic structures of our cells, among other critical functions.[173]

The thing is, we're all getting omega-3s, we're just not getting enough. At least, not enough compared to the other fatty acids we're eating, called omega-6s.

Your body evolved to function on a 1-to-1 ratio between omega-6 and omega-3 fatty acids. The average American diet has a ratio closer to 16-to-1.[174] This huge imbalance makes it more difficult for cells to take in precious nutrients—and thus makes them more susceptible to injury and inflammation.[175] In the brain, reduced cell health leads to impaired mental health.[176]

What does all this mean for your mental health? Getting the right amount, and balance, of omega-3s has a dramatic effect on inflammation and its related symptoms. In one study, just 12 weeks of omega-3 supplementation lowered not only inflammation but also anxiety and depression symptoms in young adults.[177] Funny thing: the "young adults" in that study were medical students. That's no small amount of anxiety to be addressed by a single supplement!

Taking daily omega-3 supplements can also improve mood, increase energy, and lead to clearer thinking[178]—not to mention

173 National Institutes of Health Office of Dietary Supplements, "Omega-3 Fatty Acids: Fact Sheet for Health Professionals," National Institutes of Health, last modified February 15, 2023, https://ods.od.nih.gov/factsheets/Omega3FattyAcids-HealthProfessional/.

174 A. P. Simopoulos, "The Importance of the Ratio of Omega-6/Omega-3 Essential Fatty Acids," *Biomedicine & Pharmacotherapy* 56, no. 8 (October 2002): 365–79, https://doi.org/10.1016/S0753-3322(02)00253-6.

175 James J. DiNicolantonio and James H. O'Keefe, "Importance of Maintaining a Low Omega-6/Omega-3 Ratio for Reducing Inflammation," *Open Heart* 5, no. 2 (2018): e000946, https://doi.org/10.1136/openhrt-2018-000946.

176 Klaus W. Lange, "Omega-3 Fatty Acids and Mental Health," *Global Health Journal* 4, no. 1 (March 2020): 18–30, https://doi.org/10.1016/j.glohj.2020.01.004.

177 Janice K. Kiecolt-Glaser et al., "Omega-3 Supplementation Lowers Inflammation and Anxiety in Medical Students: A Randomized Controlled Trial," *Brain, Behavior, and Immunity* 25, no. 8 (November 2011): 1725–34, https://doi.org/10.1016/j.bbi.2011.07.229.

178 Thomas Larrieu and Sophie Layé, "Food for Mood: Relevance of Nutritional Omega-3 Fatty Acids for Depression and Anxiety," *Frontiers in Physiology* 9 (2018), https://doi.org/10.3389/fphys.2018.01047.

supporting brain development in childhood and decreasing risks for ADHD, autism, bipolar disorder, and depression.[179]

As always, though, not all products are created equal. Studies have found that 2,000 mg (2 g) per day is the minimum dosage to see a change in the amount of omega-3 available in the brain.[180] Some omega-3 supplements are way below that amount. So look carefully at the dosage on the bottle and make sure you're taking enough. And like with any other medication or supplement, talk to your doctor before you add fish oil to your diet.

SOMETHING FISHY

Unfortunately, since most omega-3 supplements often come in the form of fish oil, it's possible that taking low-quality supplements can introduce rancid fish, mercury, or other harmful substances into your body. To get the most out of omega-3 and avoid these problems, make sure you're taking marine-source-derived supplements (usually from marine fish, although there are algae-derived versions for vegans). I recommend Nordic Naturals. I'm not affiliated with them in any way, but I do take their omega-3 supplements. They just have high-quality products.

RECOMMENDATIONS

Drugs and supplements can be effective, powerful, useful tools in your mental health toolbox, as long as they are promoting brain health and supporting your body's natural repair processes.

As power tools, though, both drugs and supplements can hurt as

---

179 James J. DiNicolantonio and James H. O'Keefe, "The Importance of Marine Omega-3s for Brain Development and the Prevention and Treatment of Behavior, Mood, and Other Brain Disorders," *Nutrients* 12, no. 8 (August 4, 2020): 2333, https://doi.org/10.3390/nu12082333.

180 David Mischoulon, "Omega-3 Fatty Acids for Mood Disorders," *Harvard Health Blog*, October 27, 2020, https://www.health.harvard.edu/blog/omega-3-fatty-acids-for-mood-disorders-2018080314414.

much as they help. You should know what you're taking, why you're taking it, how long you will be on it—and how your doctor will help you get off it when you're ready. You should be aware of potential side effects and how the new drug or supplement might interact with what you're already taking.

In addition to working with your healthcare provider, there are some other actions you can take to get the most out of the drugs and supplements that are out there.

GET YOUR BASELINE TESTED

Listen, I hate—hate hate *hate*—having my blood drawn. I hate it. I used to resist it with every fiber of my body. But once I discovered just how much blood testing could show me about myself and how I could feel better, I have to admit, I changed my tune. I still don't love it by any means, but I'm totally willing to get poked with a needle if it reveals this level of insight.

There are all different kinds of blood tests, and each reveals something different about your likelihood of getting certain diseases, your current levels of necessary vitamins and other healthy compounds, and your levels of inflammation.

Basic blood work should include tests for common vitamin deficiencies. Many people are deficient in key nutrients without knowing it—and many others start taking vitamins or other supplements without knowing whether they're deficient or not. Getting too much of some vitamins can be as dangerous as having too little. Find out with your doctor where your levels are, what you can manage with diet, and where supplements or drugs might help.

In general, baseline blood work will also give you information about your risk for diseases like heart disease, important body processes like kidney and immune function, and key health indicators like blood sugar level. These can point to overall health but may also indicate inflammation-related symptoms.

If you want the full picture of inflammation, you should ask for inflammatory marker testing specifically. These tests look at bio-markers for inflammation, like erythrocyte sedimentation rate (ESR), high-sensitivity C-reactive protein (hs-CRP), and interleukin-6. This kind of testing can provide a window into what's happening in your body and inform your and your doctor's choices about your care. Surprisingly, this kind of testing is not routine practice, so you may need to request it separately.

Finally, although it's less common, genetic testing looks at the unique genetic blueprint that makes you different from everyone else on earth. It can look at biomarkers that suggest you might be more or less predisposed to certain conditions that can affect your mental health, and it may open up new treatment options for you. Your doctor can advise on genetic tests that could be a good fit for you.

CREATE A STRATEGY

Once you've done your blood work (and maybe genetic testing), the next step is to sit down with your healthcare provider and create a plan. This could be your doctor, naturopath, nurse practitioner, or other clinician.

The most important thing to do at this point is ask questions: Where are your deficiencies? What supplements might help your body get the basic resources it needs to heal? Are there potential problems combining any of the drugs or supplements you want to take or are already taking? Does your genetic testing suggest a specific cause for your condition, or create potential problems with any drugs or supplements?

Everyone is different, so every plan will be different. In fact, if you get nothing else from this chapter, remember this: you are unique, your body is unique, and your situation is unique. What works for others might not work for you. Work with your healthcare provider to know what you're taking and why.

DOWNSHIFTING IMMUNE OVERDRIVE

When Ash finally went to their doctor to discuss their depression, they were at their wits' end. They just couldn't imagine taking SSRIs again, not after the side effects they had last time. But with work getting so stressful and the depression coming back, Ash didn't feel like they could get by without something to help make it through the next few months.

Fortunately, Ash's doctor ran blood work, and when Ash came back for their follow-up, the doctor talked them through it. It turned out Ash had very low vitamin D and low white blood cell counts—both signs that their immune system was working in overdrive.

The doctor suggested that he and Ash try to correct those problems before getting Ash back on the SSRIs. Over the next several months, under their doctor's supervision, Ash took vitamin D, zinc, folic acid, and B$_{12}$ supplements to correct their deficiencies and improve their baseline well-being.

Ash started to see changes after just a few weeks. Their depression lifted enough to get their work motivation back. They decided not to go back on the SSRIs quite yet. Although that option was always there, it didn't feel like they were being forced to choose between debilitating depression and almost equally bad side effects. The relief alone went a long way to helping Ash move forward.

Pharmaceuticals are very often the first recommendation for common mental health issues like depression and anxiety. But they can hurt as much as they help, and how they affect you depends a lot on your own chemistry, genetics, and life circumstances.

As Ash found, supplements can help support the body's own healing mechanisms and help get things back to baseline—as long as you know where you're deficient and how much to take.

While medications are the first type of treatment recommended for most people with depression and other mental health issues, many are also encouraged to try therapy. We're at an exciting time for therapy. State-of-the-art, evidence-based practices are offering new hope for people who are suffering, but just like with medications and supplements, not all therapy methods are created equal.

How can you know what types of therapy might actually support your brain and calm that neuroinflammation? That's the question for our next chapter.

TL;DR

→ Medication is the most common treatment for many mental health issues, including depression and anxiety. SSRIs are the most common medications for these conditions, but their effectiveness is limited.

→ It turns out the prevailing "chemical imbalance" theory of mental health only represents part of the story, and more recent research has uncovered breakthroughs about the major role of inflammation.

→ Medications have to be studied and approved by the government, but supplements don't. Be cautious when using both medications and supplements for mental health; they can have dangerous side effects.

→ There are supplements that effectively reduce inflammation, especially high concentrations of inflammation-fighting foods and nutrients like omega-3s.

→ Before you take *anything* for your mental health, always consult a medical professional. Ask *why* you are taking it, *how long* they expect you to take it, and *how* they plan to get you off of it eventually.

→ Get comprehensive blood testing done to find out whether you have deficiencies that can be addressed with supplements or medication.

CHAPTER EIGHT

———

NOT JUST TALK

Therapies to Calm Your Inner Tiger

Stephanie is standing just inside the door of her home, keys in her hand. She knows she has to pick up her son from school. Actually, she should have left ten minutes ago.

She just can't make herself do it.

Over the past few months, with the help of her nutritionist, Stephanie has changed her diet completely. Her celiac disease is largely under control, and even better, she's sleeping again. Through the night mostly. The days of being woken every few hours with fierce stomach pain are finally gone.

But there's still this ongoing, crippling problem with driving.

Every time she gets behind the wheel, the memory of the accident slams into her all over again. It's like she's there, spinning in the intersection, unable to control the car, her body hurled forward against the seatbelt. She sees the hood of the truck that T-boned her carved into the passenger door, just like she saw it that day.

Every time this happens, Stephanie seems to stop breathing. Her heart races. Her hands feel cold. She feels like she's having a heart

NOT JUST TALK · 197

attack, and even though she knows it isn't true, she can't calm herself down. The panic is like an animal living in her chest, waiting to wake up and maul her from inside whenever she crosses an intersection or sees a black pickup truck in her peripheral vision.

Recently, every time she does manage to drive herself somewhere, she returns home exhausted. She avoids the road where she had the accident, which means taking an extra 20 minutes every time her daughter goes to practice. She can see her daughter rolling her eyes in the passenger seat, but there's no way she can go back through that intersection.

The worst day was last week, when it got so bad she couldn't leave the house at all. She had to call her husband to come home from work early to pick up the kids and go to the grocery store. He didn't complain, but Stephanie knows it was a bad day for him to leave early.

She doesn't want to live like this. Dependent. Exhausted. She wants her life back.

WHAT'S GOING ON HERE?

Stephanie is clearly doing better. Her physical symptoms are largely under control. The accident was years ago. Her kids are long over it. So what's going on with her?

What Stephanie doesn't realize is that she's suffering from trauma.

The word "trauma" refers to several different things, and that can sometimes confuse people. It's a word that gets used a lot, to refer to a lot of different experiences. Oddly enough, sometimes the people who have experienced the clearest trauma are the least willing to believe their experiences "count"—even when understanding trauma would help them make sense of what's happening to them.

What Stephanie experienced when her car was hit by a pickup truck was trauma. It was a moment of extreme stress that impacted her in far-reaching, negative ways.

But it's not always as obvious as that.

Trauma occurs any time that an event, circumstance, or envi-

ronment overwhelms an individual's ability to cope with or remove themselves from the experience.

To make things more complicated, the word "trauma" also refers to the long-term, lasting effects of the event in your body or mind. Trauma is both: the event *and* how your body and mind respond to it.

Your body and mind are wired to be resilient, to handle whatever happens in the course of your day, to keep you safe and healthy. When you encounter a difficult moment in your day, stress peaks, but then it subsides again.

But sometimes an event or situation is just too much. The systems get drowned by the stress response and can't tip the balance back to normal.

As we talked about in Section One, the difficulty for modern humans is that we're disconnected from our natural ways of returning to baseline. It's not possible for modern humans to act out our natural responses to stress in most of the situations we find ourselves in. If someone acts aggressively toward you at work, you can't jump around the office and shake and yell until you feel better. Instead, even as your body screams at you internally, you sit still. Your legs tense up, you get fidgety—but you don't get up and run away.

If you've ever come home at the end of a long day and felt irritated at absolutely everything and angry at the smallest sound, that's why. You're stuck with an emotional response that never got resolved. You haven't completed the stress cycle. The stress is now living in your body.

That's why, years after her car accident, Stephanie's body is acting like it's still happening. Even though she wasn't physically injured in the collision, she still has flashbacks and panic attacks. If anything, they are getting worse. That's trauma. Her nervous system believed that she was at risk of serious injury or death, which created a cascade of stress chemicals and physical reactions.

Those reactions were never fully resolved. Her system has not been able to pull itself back to baseline. She is stuck.

That stuckness is PTSD.

THE TIGER ON YOUR SHOULDER

When I first talked about fight-or-flight and the stress response, I said it was a natural response our ancestors developed to real dangers. When there's a tiger in the forest, it's better to run first and ask questions later.

The modern world can sometimes seem like a fun-house mirror of tigers. Everything from the sounds of beeping horns and garbage trucks in the street to the constant push of deadlines and expectations activates your stress response. Even though none of them are real tigers, your system responds with stress anyway.

PTSD is a very special kind of tiger that sits on your shoulder.

It's basically a stressor that you carry around with you. When you experience trauma, your body gets stuck in fight-or-flight, and that triggers your mind to react as if there's a tiger around every corner—or behind the wheel of your car.

PTSD is commonly associated with veterans who have served in war zones or victims of abuse. But there's a wide range of situations and conditions that can cause PTSD. The initial trauma can be a single event like an injury or a drawn-out fearful situation like a toxic relationship.

When it comes to trauma and PTSD, the cause does not have to be physical. Your mind and body experience emotional stress just as powerfully as physical stress. You don't have to be physically harmed for the stress response to turn on or get stuck.

If at some point your nervous system doesn't feel safe and you're not able to take action to resolve it, that's trauma. And if you don't ever get the chance to fully clear that response, the traumatic response can build on itself and become PTSD.

Trauma is about your threshold or capacity for dealing with stress. A traumatic event or circumstance is anything that exceeds that capacity. Looking at your life experiences compassionately through this lens can be tremendously helpful and supportive.

Furthermore, that threshold is different for different people. What overwhelms your system might not affect someone else the same way—and vice versa. Genetics, childhood experiences, training, physical health, and tons of other factors can affect how someone experiences an event. (That's part of why the practices in Section Two are so important. Being well rested, eating well, and moving can make you more resilient.)

Whatever the cause, whether it's the death of a beloved pet or a challenging situation at work, if the stress is beyond your threshold or capacity to cope and rebalance, you can experience trauma.

In other words, whether you're living with trauma and PTSD doesn't just depend on what type of event or situation you've experienced. It's all about the effect the event has on your nervous system. Or, to be more accurate, your nervous systems.

THE TWO NERVOUS SYSTEMS

Understanding nervous system arousal is critical to understanding how you get "stuck" in trauma.

At the big-picture level, your nervous system has two parts: the *central nervous system* and the *peripheral nervous system*. Your central nervous system includes your brain and spinal cord, while your peripheral nervous system includes all the other parts, especially the nerves and neurons that stretch out from your spinal cord to your muscles, organs, and skin. Makes sense, right? The central nervous system is made up of the two big structures in the middle (center) of the body, and the peripheral nervous system is everything radiating out to the edges (the periphery).

These systems work together like air traffic control. Sitting in the tower, overlooking the entire system, is your brain. It communicates its decisions out to the rest of the body through the spinal cord, just like an air traffic controller uses the radio to tell planes where to land, when to take off, and so on.

But air traffic control can't work all on its own. It needs incoming information to make good decisions. That information can come from sensors out on the runways or even from the pilots themselves.

That's like the peripheral nervous system—the skin and eyes and nerves and other sensory organs—sending information back to the brain.

YOU DON'T CHOOSE STRESS

Here's where it gets a bit more complicated. The peripheral system itself has two parts: the *somatic* and the *autonomic*. The word "somatic" refers to the body, and the word "autonomic" refers to something that's unconscious. It's similar to "automatic." In general, the somatic nervous system controls voluntary movements (like raising your hand) and transmits sensory information like touch, pressure, temperature, and pain from your skin and muscles to your brain.

The autonomic nervous system, on the other hand, controls your unconscious, involuntary responses. Your breathing, heartbeat, and temperature regulation are all parts of the autonomic system. These actions occur unconsciously, without thinking about them. This part of your nervous system takes care of your most basic survival processes. After all, you don't want to have to remember to breathe!

The autonomic system is key to how stress and trauma are handled in the body. Think about what you know so far about the stress response. Heart rate increases. Breathing speeds up. Body temperature heats up. These responses are directed by the autonomic nervous system, meaning that they happen unconsciously, without you choosing how to respond.

If it had to wait for you to choose how to act, the tiger would have eaten you already. The fact that it happens automatically is the whole point. You don't get to decide whether to have a stress response to an event. Your body just goes ahead and does it.

RAMPED UP, CALMED DOWN, OR STUCK?

Here's where we get down to the nitty-gritty of the stress response in your body. Buckle up for some science here.

There are two main ways your autonomic system responds to your experiences.

The two states are called *sympathetic* and *parasympathetic*. Think of these as "amped up" versus "calmed down."

The sympathetic system is your inner superhero, leaping into action as soon as you see a threat. It's the fight-or-flight system we talked about earlier. The parasympathetic system is the opposite. When the danger is gone, your body calms down, going into "rest-and-digest" mode. These two work like a seesaw, going back and forth to keep you safe and in balance.

It's just like the Hulk. When he sees danger, he gets huge and fast and powerful, fighting off the bad guys. Then, when the danger is gone, he turns back into unassuming Bruce Banner. And just like the Hulk, you want to spend most of your time in the parasympathetic, Bruce Banner state. Look at the damage the Hulk causes. Sometimes it's necessary to save the city, but you don't want to Hulk it up all the time.

Die Hard and the Stress Response

Whenever I think about the sympathetic nervous system, I always think about *Die Hard 2*.

In case you haven't seen it, *Die Hard 2* is a Bruce Willis action thriller about a terrorist plot at an airport. It's also an amazing metaphor for how your body responds to stress.

In the movie, Willis's character breaks into the air traffic control tower to tell the higher-ups that something is wrong. Once they recognize the threat, the controllers leap into action. Suddenly, everything in the control room speeds up. The controllers are sending out messages as fast as they can.

Then the runways are closed, and planes start building up in the airspace above the airport, not able to land.

Chaos erupts. The pace of the action increases—so much so that mistakes are made. One person makes a decision, then someone else changes it. The higher-ups start reacting to incoming information without really thinking it through. One disaster after another causes damage to the airport, to the planes, to the characters themselves.

Of course, Bruce Willis saves the day. Once the event is over and everything is taken care of, the pace slows again. Cleanup starts. The higher-ups are back in charge and landing planes safely once more.

See what I mean? The sympathetic nervous system reacts a lot like that control tower. A message comes in that *something is wrong*, and the system speeds up. Heart rate, breathing, everything ratchets up to respond quickly. And as the stress continues, wires get crossed, tension rises, and the central command center starts responding to *everything* like it's an immediate threat. It becomes reactive.

But—good news—once the brain is able to calm itself and the threat is removed (thanks to your internal Bruce Willis), the parasympathetic system kicks back in and starts restoring balance.

The thing is, if your nervous system is chronically disrupted and on high alert because of trauma, you're basically living in fight-or-flight all the time. You won't turn green from being in stress all the time, but your nervous system will lose its ability to regulate between the two states.

When that happens, a small thing like a barking dog will make you jump out of your skin, or a single unhappy Slack message will get you thinking you're going to lose your job.

This state of constantly being stuck in the "on" position in the sympathetic nervous system is called *hypervigilance*. It helps create the circular, self-feeding nature of post-traumatic stress and chronic inflammation. It would be like an air traffic control center deciding to have random crash alerts *every single day*, even when there was nothing bad happening, just to stay vigilant in case of threats.

To be effective at managing the long-term, chronic effects of trauma, a therapy method has to calm your chronic sympathetic nervous system arousal and get you back into the healthy back-and-forth of stress (when appropriate) and restoration.

THE INFLAMMATION CONNECTION

The nervous system isn't the only body system that gets activated by the fight-or-flight response.

When the sympathetic nervous system is activated, the brain responds as if there's a threat. The hypothalamus signals the release of adrenaline, and the adrenal cortex releases cortisol. (Check back to Chapter Three for a refresher on the HPA axis and how hormones are activated during stress.)

When the sympathetic nervous system is activated, your body also circulates more pro-inflammatory cytokines—those messengers that tell the body to create inflammation to fight off threats. Over time, a nervous system that's constantly in sympathetic arousal creates chronic inflammation.

When you look at the overall picture of the stress response, it's no surprise that Stephanie experienced serious quality of life issues following her accident. Researchers have found that just *looking* at violent images in the news led 22 percent of the more than 1,000 participants in their study to develop symptoms associated with PTSD even though *none of them* had previous trauma. Many of them even developed difficulties in daily work and school functioning, and in social interactions following the study.[181]

The highly evolved human nervous system is not something to mess with. It was designed to protect you from harm, and by gosh it is going to protect you, even when the dangers you're facing are just on the TV. That's because the parts of the brain that respond to stress recognition and signals from the eyes and ears can't discern between a real threat and make-believe, or on-screen, images.

(Also, maybe a reason to not watch the news so much—just saying.)

Here's something else crazy: researchers can actually *see* stressful

---

181 E. Alison Holman et al., "Media Exposure to Collective Trauma, Mental Health, and Functioning: Does It Matter What You See?," *Clinical Psychological Science* 8, no. 1 (January 2020): 111–24, https://doi. org/10.1177/2167702619858300.

events in your body. What I mean is that there are biological effects of stress that can be identified and measured. Inflammation is one of those markers. When researchers have gone looking for *why*, exactly, stressful life experiences are correlated with outcomes like depression, inflammation is one of the causes they've identified.

At the same time, the stress response also suppresses immune function, changes your blood flow, and increases blood pressure. So while inflammation is running rampant, you're also more susceptible to illnesses, infections, and diseases that make your body fight even harder.[182]

It's a vicious cycle.

Fortunately, it can be paused, stopped, or even reversed. Therapies that help you switch your body from fight-or-flight back to rest-and-restore also help tackle inflammation and slow down the pro-inflammatory stress cycle.

THERAPY IS HEALTHCARE

The sad reality is that a lot of people who could be helped by these therapies are put off by the stigma around mental health. Even people who come to my brain fitness centers looking for support for mental health symptoms are sometimes ashamed or hesitant to "go to therapy" because they think it means there's something "wrong" with them.

Let me put that to rest right here. Mental healthcare is *healthcare*, like setting a broken bone or taking insulin for diabetes. Mental health issues like depression, anxiety, trauma, and fatigue are conditions that affect your quality of life and that can be improved with the help of the right team of experts. Just like any other medical condition.

Don't deny yourself access to the care you need because of stigma.

---

182 Firdaus S. Dhabhar, "Effects of Stress on Immune Function: The Good, the Bad, and the Beautiful," *Immunologic Research* 58 (2014): 193–210, https://doi.org/10.1007/s12026-014-8517-0.

BUT WHAT ABOUT TALK THERAPY?

A lot of the stigma around therapy is related to what's called *talk therapy*. It's what most of us imagine when we hear the word "therapy," and it's the cause of a lot of misconceptions about what modern therapy actually looks like.

When we think about talk therapy, we tend to imagine a stereotypical movie therapist: a gray-haired man in spectacles nodding along and taking notes while a patient lies on a couch, revealing personal stories about their life.

This image of therapy stretches all the way back to Sigmund Freud, the Austrian neurologist who founded psychoanalysis in the late 19th century. Freud believed that mental illness was caused by repressed desires and unconscious urges. His version of psychoanalysis involved the patient talking through early experiences to discover what had been suppressed.

Unfortunately, a lot of what therapists and analysts did throughout the 20th century was based on what early practitioners like Freud believed about how the mind works, without a lot of evidence that they were correct.

Don't get me wrong. Not everything those early analysts said was mistaken. But because they didn't have the technologies, tools, or research we have today, they had to base their ideas on the theories and observations they had available.

Needless to say, a lot has changed since 1896. Now there are science-driven, evidence-based therapy methods that directly address the causes and symptoms of mental illness. Even the most traditional forms of psychotherapy (the general term for talk therapy) have been studied and updated.

SO MANY OPTIONS

Let's recap. Stress leads to inflammation, which leads to quality-of-life-impacting symptoms. Therapy is one way to reduce stress and break the cycle of inflammation. Modern therapy is evidence-based healthcare, and it's nothing to feel ashamed about.

Great. Understood.

So now that you've decided to jump in and try out therapy, what's your next step? If you're anything like me, your first step for anything is to Google it. Okay, so I Google "therapy," and I get…about 400 types of therapy to choose from. That's—a lot. It's an overwhelming amount, actually.

This isn't just a scenario I'm imagining, by the way. This is exactly what happened when I was first searching for ways to tame my own mental and cognitive health challenges. My doctor recommended that I try therapy, so I decided, what the heck. My depression and fatigue were dragging me down, and I needed help.

Googling, I can tell you right now, did *not* help. There was just too much there. Too many options. I spent hundreds of hours digging into the research on all these different types of therapy, finding out which were backed by real evidence and which might work for each of my different symptoms.

The research was a slog, but what I discovered did give me hope. There *were* therapy options that could not only make me "feel better" in the short term, but could actually *retrain my nervous system* and help me return to my old self.

Perhaps the most important thing I learned was that not all therapies do the same work. Trauma, in particular, requires a specialized, expert approach.

Just like you wouldn't go to an ear-nose-and-throat doctor for a heart attack, different therapy specializations and approaches work better for different individuals, conditions, and symptoms. What is best for an eight-year-old with anxiety may not be what's most impactful for a 62-year-old with war flashbacks.

Think about shopping for clothes. You wouldn't walk into J.Crew and tell the salesperson, "I want to buy some clothes." They would need to know what kind of clothes you wanted. Do you need pants? What kind are you looking for? Are you playing pickleball or going to work?

Great questions—and very similar to the ones you'll need to ask yourself about what therapy options will work for you.

So, without any more ado, let's talk therapy. And pants.

THERAPIES THAT TAME THE TIGERS

So there you are, in the "therapy" department. You're looking through the selection, trying to find a good fit. What's available? What will work for your specific issues and symptoms?

Consider me your personal shopper. I'm not here to recommend any particular therapy, but to show you what is out there and what evidence there is for each approach.

As far as your nervous system is concerned, traumas and stresses are all tigers. And those tigers can all lead, over time, to chronic inflammation and mental health symptoms. But not all symptoms, not all traumas and stresses, and not all individuals respond to all therapies the same way. Different therapeutic approaches have been developed to cope with different tigers, so to speak.

Your job, in other words, isn't to find the "right" therapy—but the right therapy for you.

COGNITIVE BEHAVIORAL THERAPY (CBT):
THE BLUE JEANS OF THERAPY

When you're looking through the options in the therapy catalog, cognitive behavioral therapy (CBT) is that reliable and versatile standby: a good pair of blue jeans. CBT is by far the most common, most studied, and most widely available form of talk therapy today.

CBT was first developed by a psychiatrist named Aaron Beck in the 1960s. He originally focused on depression and how a depressed person's thoughts could keep them feeling depressed, even when good things happened in their lives.

The tools and methods he developed, which eventually became

known as CBT, were very effective at helping change that dynamic for depressed patients.[183]

Since then, CBT has also been shown to treat a host of other mental health conditions and symptoms, including:

- Anxiety[184]
- Phobias[185]
- PTSD[186]
- Sleep disorders[187]
- OCD[188]
- Addictions[189]
- Chronic pain[190]
- Schizophrenia[191]
- Coping after a spinal cord injury[192]

---

183 Manaswi Gautam et al., "Cognitive Behavioral Therapy for Depression," *Indian Journal of Psychiatry* 62, supplement 2 (January 2020): s223–29, https://doi.org/10.4103/psychiatry.indianjpsychiatry_772_19.

184 Antonia N. Kaczkurkin and Edna B. Foa, "Cognitive-Behavioral Therapy for Anxiety Disorders: An Update on the Empirical Evidence," *Dialogues in Clinical Neuroscience* 17, no. 3 (2015): 337–46, https://doi.org/10.31887/DCNS.2015.17.3/akaczkurkin.

185 Han-I. Wang et al., "Cost and Effectiveness of One Session Treatment (OST) for Children and Young People with Specific Phobias Compared to Multi-Session Cognitive Behavioural Therapy: Results from a Randomised Controlled Trial," *BMC Psychiatry* 22 (August 12, 2022): 547, https://doi.org/10.1186/s12888-022-04192-8.

186 Laura E. Watkins, Kelsey R. Sprang, and Barbara O. Rothbaum, "Treating PTSD: A Review of Evidence-Based Psychotherapy Interventions," *Frontiers in Behavioral Neuroscience* 12 (2018), https://doi.org/10.3389%2Ffnbeh.2018.00258.

187 Erin Koffel, Adam D. Bramoweth, and Christi S. Ulmer, "Increasing Access to and Utilization of Cognitive Behavioral Therapy for Insomnia (CBT-I): A Narrative Review," *Journal of General Internal Medicine* 33, no. 6 (2018): 955–62, https://doi.org/10.1007/s11606-018-4390-1.

188 Joseph O'Neill and Jamie D. Feusner, "Cognitive-Behavioral Therapy for Obsessive–Compulsive Disorder: Access to Treatment, Prediction of Long-Term Outcome with Neuroimaging," *Psychology Research and Behavior Management* 8 (2015): 211–23, https://doi.org/10.2147/PRBM.S75106.

189 Kathleen M. Carroll and Brian D. Kiluk, "Cognitive Behavioral Interventions for Alcohol and Drug Use Disorders: Through the Stage Model and Back Again," *Psychology of Addictive Behaviors* 31, no. 8 (2017): 847–61, https://psycnet.apa.org/doi/10.1037/adb0000311.

190 Jae-A Lim et al., "Cognitive-Behavioral Therapy for Patients with Chronic Pain," *Medicine* 97, no. 23 (June 2018): e10867, https://doi.org/10.1097%2FMD.0000000000010867.

191 Douglas Turkington et al., "Cognitive-Behavioral Therapy for Schizophrenia: A Review," *Journal of Psychiatric Practice* 10, no. 1 (January 2004): 5–16, https://doi.org/10.1097/00131746-200401000-00002.

192 Swati Mehta et al., "An Evidence-Based Review of the Effectiveness of Cognitive Behavioral Therapy for Psychosocial Issues Post-Spinal Cord Injury," *Rehabilitation Psychology* 56, no. 1 (2011): 15–25, https://psycnet.apa.org/doi/10.1037/a0022743.

(Side note: Every one of these conditions or symptoms has been considered difficult or, in some cases, nearly impossible to treat at some point. It's incredible that one approach can provide relief for so many of them.)

CBT helps people learn to replace negative thoughts and behaviors with more positive ones. Depressed people, for example, tend to have very negative interpretations of events. If someone doesn't respond to them at the office, their brain says, "That person doesn't like me." A nondepressed person, on the other hand, might think, "I guess that person didn't see me" and move on.

Shifting those negative thought patterns helps shift your emotions and perceptions, creating a positive cycle of improvement.[193]

CBT sessions can include conversation, role playing, and calming techniques and often lead to a greater sense of confidence and an improved ability to recognize and avoid problem patterns in your life.

CBT was one of the tools Stephanie used to manage her panic.

First of all, she learned to recognize her triggers. Throughout the day, she notices what situations cause her panic attacks and the negative thoughts that go with them. Once she can recognize when one of those situations is happening, she's able to challenge those thoughts and come up with different, less anxiety-provoking interpretations of what's happening.

On top of that, her CBT therapist teaches her some relaxation techniques, like deep breathing and muscle relaxation. When she gets into a panicked state, she can use these new skills to calm herself and regain a sense of control.

Finally, once she's got enough coping and managing skills to feel like she can handle it, her therapist encourages her to gradually expose herself to triggering situations like driving through the intersection where her accident happened. Every time she goes through the intersection, she uses her new skills and feels less anxiety.

---

193 Psychology Tools, "What is CBT?," accessed May 11, 2023, https://www.psychologytools.com/self-help/what-is-cbt/.

Over time, this combination of new techniques helps her manage her panic so she can go about her daily life with less anxiety. She experiences fewer triggering moments, which gives her a much higher everyday quality of life.

More than Just Talk

The important thing to remember is that CBT isn't just talking. It's talking with a practitioner who has been educated in very particular methods of guiding your conversations to develop new perspectives and change old patterns and behaviors. It's about turning your prefrontal cortex (your conscious, rational brain) into an ally to make sense of chaotic, painful, or harmful patterns or experiences in your life.

Sometimes people think that CBT is just based on the idea that talking about your problems helps you feel better. That is true—but it's more than that. You don't just "feel better." CBT has a physical effect on the brain. Sounds strange, but it's true: talking, *if it's done right*, using proven tools, can reduce the physical inflammation associated with conditions like depression, treating not only the symptoms but the underlying physical disturbance as well.[194]

In fact, the inflammation-reducing effects of the sessions are a major component in why people feel better and why CBT has a long-term effect. Research suggests that once you start feeling symptom relief from CBT, you continue to feel better over time. You don't just revert back as soon as you stop the therapy.

In one study, ten sessions of CBT reduced anxiety symptoms across the board for a group of young people—and the results still

---

194 Adrian L. Lopresti, "Cognitive Behaviour Therapy and Inflammation: A Systematic Review of Its Relationship and the Potential Implications for the Treatment of Depression," *Australian & New Zealand Journal of Psychiatry* 51, no. 6 (2017): 565–82, https://doi.org/10.1177/0004867417701996; and Bing Cao et al., "Does Cognitive Behaviour Therapy Affect Peripheral Inflammation of Depression? A Protocol for the Systematic Review and Meta-Analysis," *BMJ Open* 11, no. 12 (2021): e048162, https://doi.org/10.1136/bmjopen-2020-048162.

held up *four years later*.[195] That is a long time to feel better from one intervention.

So why does CBT work? How can talking to someone with this training actually reduce inflammation markers? There are two main reasons.

First, there is the experience of the sessions themselves. Most people with trauma and chronic inflammation, who are living with hypervigilance and constant arousal, have trouble feeling safe. When your brain never feels safe, it never shuts off the stress cycle.

Being in a guided CBT session gives you an hour of safety. An hour of feeling supported and not alone. That experience by itself is nervous-system regulating and can help nudge your system back into the rest-and-restore, self-healing mode. It interrupts the constant fight-or-flight pattern and creates a break from new stressors. This aspect of CBT can function as an acute intervention, helping you feel better right away.

Second, the skills and changes in perspective and behavior that CBT creates have direct nervous-system adjusting effects.

Not thinking in absolute terms, feeling more present in everyday life (rather than being pulled into PTSD flashbacks, for example) and not engaging in "what if" worries, among other changes, can have calming effects every day, even when you're not in a session. Over time, this calmer approach reduces your brain's fight-or-flight response, allows the HPA axis to rebalance, and lets you live better in your everyday life.

There's a reason CBT is such a popular, widely used therapy style. It's approachable and effective. But there are other types of therapy that can be important tools in your inflammation-fighting toolbox as well.

---

195 Arne Kodal et al., "Long-Term Effectiveness of Cognitive Behavioral Therapy for Youth with Anxiety Disorders," *Journal of Anxiety Disorders* 53 (January 2018): 58–67, https://doi.org/10.1016/j.janxdis.2017.11.003.

DIALECTICAL BEHAVIOR THERAPY (DBT):
THE MOTORCYCLE CRUISERS APPROACH

If CBT is a pair of everyday blue jeans—versatile and good for a lot of different occasions—then DBT is a pair of leather-reinforced motorcycle cruising pants. Cruising pants are made of tough, heavy material and protect the wearer against injury while they're on their bike. They're exactly what you need when you need them, but not what you'd pick out for daily wear.

CBT helps change your thoughts and how you react to situations. It helps you change negative thoughts into more positive ones and teaches you new ways to handle tough feelings. That could apply to almost anyone. DBT, on the other hand, gives you specific tools for handling strong emotions. It can be super helpful if your emotions sometimes feel really big and hard to control. DBT gives you techniques to calm down, understand your emotions, and communicate even in the middle of challenging situations.

"Dialectical" means finding a balance between two things that might seem opposite. People with very strong emotions, especially "negative" emotions like anger, sometimes need to learn how to accept and love themselves even while they admit that they need better ways to control their feelings. Those things might seem like opposites (accepting yourself and also wanting to change), and DBT can help you do both at once.

As a result, DBT is well tailored to the complex experiences and challenges that people with a history of traumatic experiences often face. Working with a DBT-trained practitioner can help you learn new skills to better regulate your emotions, navigate conflict with others, and reduce the impact of trauma on your everyday life.

For people living with more severe symptoms of PTSD in particular, DBT can be life-changing, even compared to other therapy approaches. Abuse and trauma suffered in childhood can be among the most difficult experiences to recover from, but the women in one study showed substantial improvements in PTSD symptoms from their weekly DBT sessions and had 20 percent higher recovery rates compared to a group of women doing a form of CBT.[196] This and other similar studies suggest that even more severe traumatic experiences can be treated with the right therapeutic approach.

Especially if you have difficulty managing emotions or are experiencing more severe symptoms like self-harm, eating disorders, or impulsive behavior, DBT is worth exploring.

THERAPY AND...FLOSSING?

Surprisingly, your mouth can say a lot about your brain health. Very recently, researchers found that depression can increase the risk of gum disease, and vice versa.[197] Gum disease is also associated with an increased risk of developing chronic diseases, including cardiovascular disease, diabetes, and respiratory disease.[198]

The common link between all of these? Inflammation.

"Poor oral health may cause declines in brain health, so we need to be extra careful with our oral hygiene because it has implications far beyond the mouth," says Dr. Cyprien Rivier, MD, MS, Yale School of Medicine.[199] Who knew brushing and flossing regularly could reduce the risk of depression and chronic diseases? It might be time to get that checkup scheduled!

196 Martin Bohus et al., "Dialectical Behavior Therapy for Posttraumatic Stress Disorder (DBT-PTSD) Compared with Cognitive Processing Therapy (CPT) in Complex Presentations of PTSD in Women Survivors of Childhood Abuse: A Randomized Clinical Trial," *JAMA Psychiatry* 77, no. 12 (2020): 1235–45, https://doi.org/10.1001/jamapsychiatry.2020.2148.

197 Alexandrina L. Dumitrescu, "Depression and Inflammatory Periodontal Disease Considerations—An Interdisciplinary Approach," *Frontiers in Psychology* 7 (March 22, 2016), https://doi.org/10.3389/fpsyg.2016.00347.

198 Dawit T. Zemedikun et al., "Burden of Chronic Diseases Associated with Periodontal Diseases: A Retrospective Cohort Study Using UK Primary Care Data," *BMJ Open* 11, no. 12 (2021): e048296, https://doi.org/10.1136/bmjopen-2020-048296.

199 American Stroke Association, "Poor Oral Health May Contribute to Declines in Brain Health," news release, American Heart Association, February 2, 2023, https://newsroom.heart.org/news/poor-oral-health-may-contribute-to-declines-in-brain-health.

EYE MOVEMENT DESENSITIZATION AND REPROCESSING (EMDR): THERAPY'S SPORTY LEGGINGS

The first time I heard about EMDR, I have to admit, I was skeptical. Moving your eyes around to resolve trauma? It seemed far fetched.

But the evidence is in. Strange as it might sound, EMDR, or Eye Movement Desensitization and Reprocessing, can help your brain get unstuck—it just works in a very specific and focused way. Like your best pair of sporty leggings, EMDR gives you exactly what you need to get moving. When you want to go to the gym or a yoga class, you pull on your athletic wear, right? They're usually quick and easy to pull on and go. For a lot of people, EMDR works the same way. It can help you feel better fast, relieving your symptoms so you can do the deeper work of processing trauma and moving forward in your life.

EMDR was developed by psychologist Francine Shapiro in 1987 while she was taking a walk in the park and reflecting on some of her distressing personal memories. She noticed that as she moved her eyes, the negative emotions she was experiencing seemed to decrease. That's really how it started. Moving her eyes while she thought about her negative experiences made her feel better. That's not all there is to EMDR, but that was the origin. Shapiro's insight in the park led her to further experimentation with this technique, and eventually EMDR was born.[200]

So, yeah. It sounds a bit...unlikely. Partly because it sounds so odd, a ton of research has been done on EMDR already. And it works. EMDR significantly reduces the symptoms of PTSD, depression, anxiety, and subjective distress in PTSD patients[201]—and it is effective faster than CBT, which addresses similar types of symptoms. It is

---

200 EMDR Institute, Inc., "The History of EMDR Therapy," accessed May 14, 2023, https://www.emdr.com/history-of-emdr/.

201 Ying-Ren Chen et al., "Efficacy of Eye-Movement Desensitization and Reprocessing for Patients with Posttraumatic-Stress Disorder: A Meta-Analysis of Randomized Controlled Trials," *PLoS One* 9, no. 8 (2014): e103676, https://doi.org/10.1371%2Fjournal.pone.0103676.

also effective for generalized anxiety and a number of other mental health issues.[202]

Though there haven't yet been studies done directly on EMDR's effect on inflammation in the body, research has shown that PTSD is associated with dysregulation of the HPA axis, and EMDR therapy has been found to regulate the HPA axis in patients with PTSD.[203]

But really, why it works is less important than the fact that it *does* work. A lot of trained practitioners these days are combining EMDR with other therapies, like CBT, because it helps relieve symptoms quickly. Others offer focused sessions of EMDR by itself. Either way, it can be a powerful tool in your toolbox, especially for PTSD and related symptoms.

SOMATIC EXPERIENCING (SE): YOUR FAVORITE SWEATPANTS

Somatic Experiencing (SE) therapy focuses on changing how you physically experience post-traumatic symptoms. Your internal experience of your body is called *interoception*. It's like perception, but directed inward. If you close your eyes and concentrate, you might be able to feel your heart beating or sense that you're hungry. Those are elements of interoception.

SE therapy works because trauma doesn't just affect your brain. Traumatic experiences overwhelm your body's stress-regulation systems. As a result, many people experience trauma as internal body sensations like tension, anxiety, and even chronic pain. SE therapy acts on your interoceptive experience of your body, directly

202 Elisa Faretta and Mariella Dal Farra, "Efficacy of EMDR Therapy for Anxiety Disorders," *Journal of EMDR Practice and Research* 13, no. 4 (November 2019): 325–32, http://dx.doi.org/10.1891/1933-3196.13.4.325; and Charles Scelles and Luis Carlo Bulnes, "EMDR As Treatment Option for Conditions Other Than PTSD: A Systematic Review," *Frontiers in Psychology* 12 (September 19, 2021), https://doi.org/10.3389/fpsyg.2021.644369.

203 Sarah Schumacher et al., "Psychotherapeutic Treatment and HPA Axis Regulation in Posttraumatic Stress Disorder: A Systematic Review and Meta-Analysis," *Psychoneuroendocrinology* 98 (December 2018): 186–201, https://doi.org/10.1016/j.psyneuen.2018.08.006.

addressing the physical sensations and symptoms associated with trauma.[204]

It's like slipping into your favorite comfy sweatpants. When you get home from work, stressed and tired, and put on your sweatpants, you already feel better. Your body relaxes, and you're able to do what needs to be done. Similarly, when you release or reduce the physical symptoms and reactivity in your body, your brain has a better chance to heal.

During an SE session, the therapist will guide you to focus on your body, specifically on the physical sensations you're experiencing. The goal is to help you navigate sensations and emotions and to work to regulate the nervous system to resolve symptoms from chronic and traumatic stress. Sometimes breathing techniques are used, along with gentle touch on the arms and back. Together, these techniques help shift the nervous system's response to stress, reducing reactivity and increasing well-being.[205]

One study showed that something as simple as a hand placed on the lower back, near the kidneys, reduced heart rate and soothed participants out of fight-or-flight mode. It even worked if the participants did the touching practice themselves.[206]

One of the most important benefits of SE is its impact on resilience. Many people with PTSD experience what's called *dysregulation*. Dysregulation means it's hard for you to manage tough emotions like anger, fear, or panic. It can look like overreacting to minor negative events during the day or jumping every time you hear a noise. Resilience is the opposite: the ability to bounce back. Because SE

---

204 Marie Kuhfuss et al., "Somatic Experiencing—Effectiveness and Key Factors of a Body-Oriented Trauma Therapy: A Scoping Literature Review," *European Journal of Psychotraumatology* 12, no. 1 (2021), https://doi.org/10.1080/20008198.2021.1929023.

205 Peter Payne, Peter A. Levine, and Mardi A. Crane-Godreau, "Somatic Experiencing: Using Interoception and Proprioception as Core Elements of Trauma Therapy," *Frontiers in Psychology* 6 (February 2015), https://doi.org/10.3389/fpsyg.2015.00093.

206 Chigusa Theresa Yachi, Taichi Hitomi, and Hajime Yamaguchi, "Two Experiments on the Psychological and Physiological Effects of Touching—Effect of Touching on the HPA-Axis Related Parts of the Body on Both Healthy and Traumatized Experiment Participants," *Behavioral Sciences* 8, no. 10 (October 17, 2018): 95, https://doi.org/10.3390/bs8100095.

works directly on physical, felt experiences, it can be very effective at treating dysregulation and improving resilience.[207]

For someone who's been living in the "red zone," experiencing extreme emotions or fighting to stay in control, this can be like getting an entirely new lease on life—suddenly able to withstand the normal stressors of everyday life and interact more positively with others.

Tetris for PTSD?

Sometimes the most effective therapy...well, doesn't look a lot like therapy at all.

Even games like Tetris have been shown to prevent the onset of PTSD. In 2017, researchers at Oxford University set up computers in the emergency room. Half the people who came into the ER who had been in serious car accidents were asked to play Tetris for 20 minutes. At their one-week follow-up, the Tetris-playing group had almost 40 percent fewer intrusive memories than the control group.[208]

That's because the memories that we make while we're seeing and doing something (like driving a car in a high-stress situation) lock into a specific part of our brains during sleep, as we discussed in Chapter Six. If we use the same part of the brain to create a competing memory, like seeing Tetris blocks and focusing on putting them in specific places, that takes up space that would otherwise be used to lock in a traumatic memory of the event.

Focused activity takes up your visual bandwidth so the memories don't stick in your mind.

What's the takeaway? There are super-practical, easy-to-implement behavioral interventions that can minimize trauma-related disorders

---

207 Neal E. Winblad, Michael Changaris, and Phyllis K. Stein, "Effect of Somatic Experiencing Resiliency-Based Trauma Treatment Training on Quality of Life and Psychological Health as Potential Markers of Resilience in Treating Professionals," *Frontiers in Neuroscience* 12 (February 15, 2018), https://doi.org/10.3389/fnins.2018.00070.

208 L. Iyadurai et al., "Preventing Intrusive Memories after Trauma via a Brief Intervention Involving Tetris Computer Game Play in the Emergency Department: A Proof-of-Concept Randomized Controlled Trial," *Molecular Psychiatry* 23 (March 2018): 674–82, https://doi.org/10.1038/mp.2017.23.

and their effects...i.e., inflammation. You can't necessarily prevent a car accident, but this kind of intervention can significantly reduce the long-term aftermath.

RECOMMENDATIONS

There's a reason therapy is one of the two most common recommendations for people living with mental health issues. Any form of certified mental health support will help balance your nervous system and improve mental health.

However, approaches that directly affect the nervous system can address inflammation and other physiological aspects of mental health more quickly. When you work with your doctor or search for therapy approaches, consider those that have been proven to reduce sympathetic nervous system activation.

And for many people living with mental health issues, trauma is likely to be an issue. Look for therapies that have been designed or shown to help relieve the symptoms of trauma—and therapists who are trained to handle it.

DON'T STIGMATIZE YOURSELF

If you had heart disease, you wouldn't be ashamed to go to a cardiologist. If you broke your leg, you would go to the emergency room. Mental health may not always be seen as the equivalent of physical health, but it is. You need both to function well and live your life. Also, therapists are professionally required to keep your sessions confidential, so no one will find out you're seeing a therapist unless you tell them.

Seek the help you need, and don't worry what other people might think. You might be pleasantly surprised by the positivity and support of those around you.

FIND A LICENSED THERAPIST

Methods like CBT, DBT, and EMDR apply techniques that therapists must be specially trained to deliver. Just like you'd seek out a certified physical therapist if you tore your shoulder, you should seek out a registered clinical counselor or psychotherapist for your mental health treatment.

A coach or unlicensed counselor might be a great choice for picking a new career path, but mental health is complex and requires special training to treat. Your well-being and recovery are far too important to trust to someone without the right credentials. Any reputable therapist will be more than happy to share their education, training, and experience with you before you start working together.

If you're not sure where to start, check out PsychologyToday. com (at least if you're in the US or Canada). The site offers a list of licensed therapists whose credentials have already been reviewed, and you can filter by location, insurance provider, training, and so on. You'll get to see a quick bio and find out how to contact each provider. Additionally, online services like Talkspace and BetterHelp offer certified providers. You can also think about asking friends and family for recommendations.

LOOK FOR FIT

Just like with any relationship, there are great and not-so-great "fits" between patients and therapists. Even if someone has the qualifications and training you want, you might just not get along or feel right with them.

Therapy, especially therapy for trauma, is incredibly sensitive and personal. You have to feel safe, comfortable, and supported in the relationship. You should feel that your therapist understands your issues, sees you for who you are, and offers you the kind of help and support you need. There may be times when therapy is difficult, but it should never feel unsafe. You should always be able to trust your therapist to have your best interests in mind.

It can be a big leap to reach out to multiple therapists and see who feels right to you. But remember, you are investing time, effort, and money into your own personal well-being. It just makes sense to find someone who will make that investment worthwhile. The time you spend finding the right person will pay off many times over.

FINALLY SEEING PROGRESS

Eventually, Stephanie found herself almost unable to drive at all. Every time she got in the car, her whole body would shake. When she approached an intersection, she would find herself sweating, her heart pounding.

She decided that she needed more than nutrition changes. At first, she was afraid to discuss the possibility with her husband and kids. What if they judged her? What if they thought she should just "get over it"? As it turned out, they were very supportive. They wanted her to feel better.

After pursuing CBT for awhile and getting a benefit, her therapist told her about PTSD. Stephanie was surprised to find out that people with PTSD also often get autoimmune disorders like celiac disease! She hadn't realized the two things could be related.

Her CBT therapist also suggested that she try EMDR. It seemed a little strange at first, but her therapist thought it could help her make progress with her intrusive memories and anxiety.

She agreed. Her therapist gave her a recommendation for a trained practitioner at a local clinic, so she set up an appointment.

Stephanie is now two months into regular EMDR sessions, and she's already noticed that she's having fewer flashbacks. Just the other day she ran errands without having to fight back a panic attack. It was the first time she'd driven anywhere since the accident without even thinking about it. The relief was so strong she almost cried.

There is still anxiety. She still has moments of panic and triggers around driving in certain neighborhoods. But most days, she can get through her day without a panic attack, and she rarely has to ask her husband to take over for her. Even her kids have mentioned how much better she seems.

It's starting to feel like she will make it through this.

Drugs, supplements, and therapy can help a lot of people. They're usually the recommendations you're going to get from your doctor, and they are often a good place to start.

But what about those other options you might have heard about? What about your Facebook friend who keeps posting videos of herself doing yoga with goats? She says it's helped her anxiety. Could that possibly be true?

As someone who regularly plunges my body into freezing cold water for my mental health, I can tell you that some of the so-called "alternative" practices out there really do work...but not all of them. Some are backed by decades of research. Others are flash-in-the-pan social media fads.

The next chapter will explore how to tell the difference—and how you can add the most effective ones to your brain-health toolbox.

TL;DR

→ After medication, therapy is the most common approach to treating mental health issues of all kinds. It can be an important tool in your brain-health tool kit.

→ Your nervous system has two main states of being: the *sympathetic* nervous system response (the fight-or-flight response) and the *parasympathetic* nervous system response (the calm, rest-and-digest response).

→ The most effective therapy approaches are those that actually reduce the fight-or-flight and chronic stress responses in the body. By addressing stress in the nervous system, they also reduce inflammation and its related symptoms.

→ Some therapy approaches, like those outlined in this chapter, have strong evidence to support their effects on the nervous system. Take the time to research what type of therapy you need, and be sure you're working with a professional who is trained to treat your particular issues and symptoms.

CHAPTER NINE

ALTERNATIVE AND COMPLEMENTARY PRACTICES

What's "Woo-Woo" and What's Real

Jadyn just doesn't seem to be getting any better. He keeps thinking that his post-COVID-19 symptoms will go away eventually, but it isn't happening.

Learning anything new is especially hard. His short-term memory can't hold onto information like it used to, and he finds himself unable to pay attention to anything for longer than a few minutes. Plus, he's still got almost no energy, and he's feeling down and anxious.

He managed to push himself hard and get through his coding boot camp. But now he's worried that he'll lose not only his barista job, but his chance at a new career. He's afraid that COVID-19 might have been a turning point. That he might never get back to his old self.

He tries to keep himself positive, but it's hard.

Eventually, when he realizes the symptoms probably aren't going to go away on their own, Jadyn takes a day off and goes to see his doctor. The doctor runs blood work that includes inflammatory and immune markers, as well as vitamin tests.

It turns out Jadyn's immune system is in overdrive. COVID-19 put the immune system in motion, and it hasn't shut off properly, and now his blood work suggests there is systemic inflammation. The doctor tells him that he needs to eliminate as much stress as he can. Any stress will drag on the little energy he has and keep his immune system in high gear.

At first, the doctor asks if Jadyn can stop working, but that's not possible. Instead, they agree that Jadyn will pause his search for a new coding job and focus on getting healthy.

The doctor suggests some things to try out, but Jadyn is skeptical. Acupuncture? Meditation? It all sounds kind of weird and not like anything he would normally do. But at this point, he's willing to try anything that might help.

The problem is, when he goes online, he just gets more confused. There are a lot of articles and ads and opinions, but it's not clear which stress relief practices actually work. He wants to do the work, but it's hard to know where to start.

SCIENCE...OR SOCIAL MEDIA?

Jadyn ran into something that I've seen time and again. When he tried to find out how to reduce his stress so his immune system could recover, he found so much information that it was almost worse than no information at all.

Practices that relieve stress and help calm the immune response are definitely out there, but as Jadyn discovered, it can be hard to know which ones really do what they claim.

So before we get to the rest of the chapter, let's take a second for a quick quiz.

POP QUIZ

Which of the following popular practices has been proven, through research, to measurably reduce markers of stress and inflammation?

Tai Chi	Forest bathing	Cold plunging	Yoga
Meditation	Breath work	Sensory deprivation	Acupuncture

Are you ready for the surprise answer?

It's all of them. There's strong research to support the benefits of every one of these practices.

But there is also a lot of noise out there. You can find someone on social media promoting almost any kind of method, whether it's 10,000 years old or was just invented yesterday. Just because a practice is talked about a lot, or is mentioned by someone influential or famous, or has a big ad budget behind it, doesn't mean it works.

Unfortunately, that leaves a lot of people in Jadyn's situation: confused, not sure where to start, and skeptical of every option.

Especially when some of this stuff can seem a bit, well, *strange*. Plunging your body into freezing cold water? Ugh, why?

The answer lies in the connection between stress, inflammation, and immune function. As you already know, stress can kick on the immune response. And if it's not turned off, it can lead to chronic inflammation and its related mental health symptoms.

Remember, too, your brain can't really tell the difference between emotional or imagined distress and physical or real-life distress. Ruminating on past experiences or imagining scary futures can turn on the stress cycle just as much as a "real" stressor. Imagined or remembered stresses can even be worse because there's nothing you can do about them. If someone yells at you, you can walk away. But if your brain keeps running a loop of someone yelling at you, there's nowhere to run.

In other words, stress isn't just something that happens around us or to us. Constant noise from a construction site next door can cause stress, absolutely. But if you've ever gone on vacation and found yourself lying next to the pool, unable to relax or enjoy yourself because of something you said at work two weeks ago—that's stress too.

The good news is that there are a lot of ways to start getting better.

ALTERNATIVE AND COMPLEMENTARY

The word *alternative* means "instead of," and the word *complementary* means "in addition to." So when someone talks about alternative medicine, they're suggesting that you might do those things *instead of* traditional Western methods like taking medicine or working with a therapist.

I prefer the term *complementary* because most of these practices won't be enough to get rid of chronic inflammation or mental health issues on their own. They're best used alongside medical treatment, therapy, or some of the more powerful "accelerator" methods I'll outline in later chapters.

Before we get into specific methods, though, let's talk for a minute about a question that scientists have just recently been getting to the bottom of. What, exactly, is your brain doing when it doesn't seem to be doing anything at all?

And what does that have to do with stress, inflammation, and mental health?

LIVING IN THE DEFAULT MODE

No single part of your brain works all by itself. Different regions work together in what are called "networks."

The two main networks are called the DMN and the WMN: the *default mode network* and the *working memory network*. When you're focused on something and actively engaged, you're in the WMN. You're "working."

When you zone out and let your mind wander, you're in the DMN, or in "default."

"Default mode" might sound like a science fiction movie or an '80s band, but the DMN is critical to your self-concept and self-awareness. It also plays a huge role in stress and depression.

The DMN comes on when you're daydreaming or your mind is wandering. Another way to think of it is that the DMN is active when you're disconnected from the present moment. You might be thinking about the past or imagining the future. Or you might be reflecting on yourself or your personality. These mental behaviors aren't connected to any particular task or activity in the present, and they're not intentionally being directed by you. Instead, they involve your mind wandering around in its own thoughts.

Throughout the day, your brain switches back and forth between WMN and DMN thought patterns. That's normal.

Without the DMN, you wouldn't be able to remember or make sense of your past experiences. You wouldn't be able to picture the future or make plans. You would have no connected sense of yourself as an individual. You would have trouble learning from mistakes and avoiding future problems.

But recent research shows that very high or constant activation of the DMN is also correlated with self-criticism and with negative mental health outcomes like anxiety and depression.[209]

The negative kind of DMN overactivity leads to rumination. To *ruminate* means "to chew over." Psychologists use it to refer to going over the same thoughts again and again. You might be thinking about the past, like replaying over and over that time you made a bad joke at a client meeting and the boss glared at you. Or you might be imagining the future, like thinking about the vacation that's coming up and picturing everything that could go wrong.

What's interesting is that everybody's "default mode" is different. That's because the thoughts you think most often are the ones that

---

209 Susan Whitfield-Gabrieli and Judith M. Ford, "Default Mode Network Activity and Connectivity in Psychopathology," *Annual Review of Clinical Psychology* 8 (April 2012): 49–76, https://doi.org/10.1146/annurev-clinpsy-032511-143049.

become your own default. If you're often worrying about the past (like people with PTSD do), then as soon as you go into the DMN state, your brain "defaults" into those thoughts about the past.

If you're always worrying about what could go wrong in the future (like people with anxiety tend to do), you'll slip into those thoughts as soon as you're not actively engaged in a task.

Certain thought patterns then become your personal default, activating as soon as you let your mind wander. And the patterns that you default to can be influenced by trauma and mental health issues. There's even evidence that childhood trauma can change an individual's DMN patterns, leading to difficulties regulating emotions and more likelihood of developing mental health issues later in life.[210]

The good news is that activities or practices that push you out of DMN patterns can substantially improve mental health and cognitive functioning.

THE INFLAMMATION CONNECTION

What does all this have to do with yoga? Or with inflammation, for that matter?

Well, we know that stress triggers an immune response: inflammation. And being *stuck in stress* means you're *stuck in inflammation*. In other words...chronic inflammation.

We also know that stress not only pushes up DMN activation, but makes it harder to turn off, so you get stuck in rumination and stressful thought-loops.[211]

People who are already struggling with mental health challenges

---

210 Tian Tian et al., "Default Mode Network Alterations Induced by Childhood Trauma Correlate with Emotional Function and SLC6A4 Expression," *Frontiers in Psychiatry* 12 (January 26, 2022), https://doi.org/10.3389/fpsyt.2021.760411; and Ruth A. Lanius, Braeden A. Terpou, and Margaret C. McKinnon, "The Sense of Self in the Aftermath of Trauma: Lessons from the Default Mode Network in Posttraumatic Stress Disorder," *European Journal of Psychotraumatology* 11, no. 1 (2020): 1807703, https://doi.org/10.1080/20008198.2020.1807703.

211 José Miguel Soares et al., "Stress Impact on Resting State Brain Networks," *PLoS One* 8, no. 6 (June 19, 2013): e66500, https://doi.org/10.1371/journal.pone.0066500.

tend to have higher DMN activation.[212] Add stress, and it becomes more and more difficult to get out of that state.

Getting out of the DMN in the moment can break your mind's hold on you, releasing you from its ruminations. It's the equivalent of walking away from the person yelling at you. Only in this case, you're finding ways to "walk away from," or switch out of, your brain's stressful default settings.

So: reduce stress, reduce inflammation. Sounds simple. It's just the small matter of *how*, exactly, to go about reducing stress. Which of the hundreds of "tips and tricks" you've seen online really work?

Turns out, it has a lot to do with attention.

TAKE BACK YOUR MIND

If your DMN is active when you're not paying attention, it makes sense that focusing and making yourself pay attention can help. You can do that in one of two ways: by putting yourself in a situation that grabs your attention from the outside, or by actively focusing your mind yourself so that you can't ruminate.

Cold plunging, for example, tends to pull people directly into the present moment. It grabs your attention and forces you to pay attention. It's pretty much impossible to ruminate when you're hit with a shock of icy water!

Meditation, on the other hand, encourages you to focus your own attention. It's not grabbing your attention from the outside but training you to seize your own attention from within. This kind of focus can also pull you out of the DMN and reduce rumination, although it can take more time to learn.

You might refer to these as *passive* and *active* practices.

These approaches tend to turn traditional thinking about the brain

---

212 Gaelle E. Doucet et al., "Transdiagnostic and Disease-Specific Abnormalities in the Default-Mode Network Hubs in Psychiatric Disorders: A Meta-Analysis of Resting-State Functional Imaging Studies," *European Psychiatry* 63, no. 1 (2020): e57, https://doi.org/10.1192/j.eurpsy.2020.57.

and mental health on its head. The traditional belief is that the brain makes decisions, and these decisions are sent out to the body, which acts out the brain's instructions.

But the brain-body connection works the other way too. Making changes in your body can change your thoughts, decisions, and emotions.

I've talked a lot about how the brain senses a danger signal and immediately turns on the fight-or-flight response, causing your heart rate to speed up, your breathing to turn shallow, and your blood vessels to narrow in key parts of your brain. With practice, though, you can consciously push this process into reverse. If you actively slow your heart rate, deepen your breathing, and restore your blood flow, your brain gets the message that it's not under stress or danger anymore—*even if the external situation hasn't changed.*

That is potentially game-changing news when your brain is constantly telling you that you're in danger when you're not. People living with trauma and PTSD, depression, anxiety, and other mental health issues are often in a fight-or-flight state even when there is no objective danger. The practices in this chapter give you the power to flip the script. You can use your body to change your mind.

What's even more amazing is that people who regularly do the kinds of practices we're going to talk about here may actually change at the genetic level.

In 2022, a research team followed a group of participants at a month-long meditation retreat. They compared the inflammatory markers of these participants to those of a group of similar people living their everyday lives. What they found is that not only did inflammation reduce in the retreat group, but the *genes that regulate inflammation themselves changed.*[213] There seems to be a single protein that acts as a kind of "on" switch for certain inflammation

---

213 María Jesús Álvarez-López et al., "Changes in the Expression of Inflammatory and Epigenetic-Modulatory Genes after an Intensive Meditation Retreat," *Comprehensive Psychoneuroendocrinology* 11 (August 2022): 100152, https://doi.org/10.1016/j.cpnec.2022.100152.

genes, and it is much less active in the people who apply mind-body practices.[214]

Needless to say, turning off stress at the genetic level can have very positive, long-term effects on your well-being.

A WALK IN THE PARK

One of the things I love best about my neighborhood is the big park that's just a few blocks from my house. I try to get out there every morning for at least a brisk walk, but as much as I love getting some movement in, what I really enjoy about the park is people watching.

The park attracts all kinds of people, many of them doing things to be healthier. It's a real inspiration to see all the different ways people are working to improve their lives.

If I get over there early enough, I see the Tai Chi club. They're out almost every morning in a big, open, grassy field to one side of the park, flowing through slow movements, sliding their feet, swooping their arms. It looks like fun, and I'm amazed by how many of them seem to be in their 70s or 80s or even older.

Later in the morning, if I'm not quite up with the Tai Chi crowd, I catch the volunteers at the neighborhood shared garden. I can almost feel the soil in my hands and the sun on my back, seeing them at work bringing food to life to share with the community. They seem to get as much from the camaraderie as they do from the gardening itself.

Some days, there are a bunch of yogis on mats in front of the lake, or one or two people sitting with their eyes closed, deep in meditation under the trees that meander through the center of the park. Once I saw a middle-aged woman in a big sun hat wandering slowly through the forested area, stopping occasionally to touch a

---

214 Ivana Buric et al., "What Is the Molecular Signature of Mind–Body Interventions? A Systematic Review of Gene Expression Changes Induced by Meditation and Related Practices," *Frontiers in Immunology* 8 (June 15, 2017), https://doi.org/10.3389/fimmu.2017.00670.

tree or look up into the swaying branches. She seemed so calm and focused that I relaxed just watching her.

Probably my favorite part of walking in the park is seeing that some of these effective, mental-health-supporting practices are gaining popularity.

As you well know by this point, the fact that someone else is doing something doesn't mean it works or that it will work for you. On the flip side, just because something sounds weird (or you don't know anyone who does it) doesn't mean you should discount it.

To help you make good choices about which alternative and complementary practices to try, I've gathered the evidence here in one place. This chapter doesn't cover every single practice that could possibly be helpful, but it gives you a lot of options to try—with the assurance that these options are all evidence-backed and useful in fighting inflammation, reducing stress, and improving your quality of life.

So...come take a walk with me. Let's see what all is out there.

DOWN DOG, DOWN WITH INFLAMMATION

I'm always impressed when I watch people doing yoga. It's like a slow ballet, a choreographed combination of physical movement and mental focus. Seeing people who can put their leg behind their head is always...interesting. But that's not at all the point.

Even the most basic yoga practice is designed to do one thing: focus your attention on the precise, practiced movements of your body. That's prime DMN-lowering activity. And it works.

One of the exciting things about yoga is that it works on its own, but it also works really well as a complementary practice—alongside other treatments. Researchers have looked at yoga therapy by itself and yoga therapy along with antidepressants, compared against antidepressants only. They looked at the effects of these therapies on brain-derived neurotrophic factor (BDNF), which we talked about earlier as a key factor in neuroplasticity and neuroinflammation.

Both the yoga groups showed significant improvement in depression scores, increased BDNF levels, and reduced levels of the stress hormone cortisol.[215]

And it's not just that yoga is "relaxing." Yoga has demonstrated anti-inflammation and anti-stress powers even compared to other popular methods such as stress-reduction education and listening to relaxing music.[216]

Short version? Yoga has it all. Increases in neuroplasticity? Check. Reduction in stress hormones? Check. Reduction in specific neuroinflammation markers? Check.[217]

So don't worry if you can't touch your toes, much less bend your leg around behind your head. Any yoga practice that helps you focus actively on your body, movement, and breath can help break you out of the stress cycle and quiet the DMN.

MEDITATION AND MINDFULNESS

When I used to think about meditation, I thought it meant trying to sit cross-legged in my living room in silence with my eyes closed and my mind clear for minutes on end. I couldn't see how being able to do that would affect my chronic work stress. Thankfully I was wrong on both counts.

Meditation refers to a broad range of practices that involve training the mind, typically to focus the attention. Doing it regularly not only reduces the magnitude of our stress and inflammatory responses inside our bodies, but on the *outside* too.

---

215 Carolina Estevao, "The Role of Yoga in Inflammatory Markers," *Brain, Behavior, & Immunity—Health* 20 (March 2022): 100421, https://doi.org/10.1016/j.bbih.2022.100421.

216 Nicole R. Nugent et al., "Benefits of Yoga on IL-6: Findings from a Randomized Controlled Trial of Yoga for Depression," *Behavioral Medicine* 47, no. 1 (2021): 21–30, https://doi.org/10.1080/08964289.2019 .1604489; and H. Lavretsky et al., "A Pilot Study of Yogic Meditation for Family Dementia Caregivers with Depressive Symptoms: Effects on Mental Health, Cognition, and Telomerase Activity," *International Journal of Geriatric Psychiatry* 28, no. 1 (January 2013): 57–65, https://doi.org/10.1002/gps.3790.

217 G. H. Naveen et al., "Serum Cortisol and BDNF in Patients with Major Depression—Effect of Yoga," *International Review of Psychiatry* 28, no. 3 (2016): 273–78, https://doi.org/10.1080/09540261.2016.11 75419.

This was demonstrated when researchers placed a hot paste on the arms of people who had meditated for years, and measured both their stress hormones and the size of the redness on their arm. Compared to people who hadn't meditated, this group had lower stress hormones, less of a brain inflammation response, and even a smaller area of red skin! They also perceived the experiment as less stressful emotionally.[218]

And that doesn't just show the power of meditation. It reminds us how closely our stress levels are connected to our body's direct, physical inflammation response.

MIND OVER DEFAULT MODE

Many meditation practices use an approach called *mindfulness*. I love mindfulness because it's something you can practice anytime, anywhere.

Let's give it a try.

Take a minute and focus on your breath. Feel it moving in and out of your nose. Let your attention narrow down, just to your breath. Hear it. Notice its warmth and the slight sensation in your chest as it rises and falls. Let the world become nothing but your breath. You can even close your eyes to block out everything else.

Go ahead. Try it.

That, at its most basic, is what mindfulness means. You could pay mindful attention to cutting up an apple or folding clothes—or you can do whole mindfulness meditation practices by yourself or with a class.

---

218 Melissa A. Rosenkranz et al., "Reduced Stress and Inflammatory Responsiveness in Experienced Meditators Compared to a Matched Healthy Control Group," *Psychoneuroendocrinology* 68 (June 2016): 117–25, https://doi.org/10.1016/j.psyneuen.2016.02.013.

Whether as part of a meditation session or not, mindfulness can be a quick way to get out of the DMN and become present and focused. It can be surprising how quickly you feel a sense of safety and calm.

A 2016 study that compared a three-day mindfulness meditation program against a basic relaxation program for stressed adult job seekers showed lower levels of inflammation markers in the mindfulness group than in the relaxation-only group, even four months later. The researchers also found the mindfulness group's DMN activity changed in a way that likely improved their emotional regulation and stress resilience.[219] Even while they were in the middle of dealing with the stress of looking for a new job, these people reduced the impact of that stress on their bodies and their brains using techniques like mindful eating, body awareness exercises, and meditation.

A little meditation goes a long way. A *single* mindfulness-based stress reduction class has been shown to create a significant improvement in both stress hormones and inflammation for a group of people with anxiety disorders.[220]

One. Class. That's not a lot of investment for such a powerful effect.

The key is to start with short, guided sessions. Just try three to five minutes at first. It's like building a new muscle, only instead of a bicep or a hamstring, this is the muscle of focus. Specifically, both meditation and mindfulness build the "muscle" of focusing on the here and now, and that does take practice. And there are great podcasts, apps, and YouTube videos that make it easy to start.

219 J. David Creswell et al., "Alterations in Resting-State Functional Connectivity Link Mindfulness Meditation with Reduced Interleukin-6: A Randomized Controlled Trial," *Biological Psychiatry* 80, no. 1 (July 1, 2016): 53–61, https://doi.org/10.1016/j.biopsych.2016.01.008.

220 Elizabeth A. Hoge et al., "The Effect of Mindfulness Meditation Training on Biological Acute Stress Responses in Generalized Anxiety Disorder," *Psychiatry Research* 262 (April 2018): 328–32, https://doi.org/10.1016/j.psychres.2017.01.006.

THANKS FOR FEELING BETTER

Here's one that surprised me: being grateful can improve your health.

One study found that people with early-stage heart failure (a disease that's strongly linked to inflammation) could reduce their inflammation just by writing down what they were grateful for. Half the participants kept a gratitude journal for eight weeks, writing down three to five big or little things they were grateful for each day. The other group got their regular treatment, but no journaling.

After the eight weeks, the people who kept journals had reduced levels of inflammation compared to the regular treatment group.[221]

Talk about something to be grateful for!

ACUPUNCTURE

Acupuncture can sometimes be a hard sell because (and I get it)... needles.

Rest assured, though, that acupuncture needles are *nothing* like the needles your doctor uses to give you a shot. They're so thin and flexible that many people report not being able to feel them at all.

And given the benefits, acupuncture might be worth getting over that fear. (Just keep in mind that unlike some of the other practices in this chapter, acupuncture requires a trained professional and isn't always cheap!)

Acupuncture has been shown to improve both cognitive impairment and markers of inflammation in people with dementia.[222] A

---

221 Laura S. Redwine et al., "Pilot Randomized Study of a Gratitude Journaling Intervention on Heart Rate Variability and Inflammatory Biomarkers in Patients with Stage B Heart Failure," *Psychosomatic Medicine* 78, no. 6 (July/August 2016): 667–76, https://doi.org/10.1097/psy.0000000000000316.

222 Jianchun Yu et al., "Effect of Acupuncture Treatment on Vascular Dementia," *Neurological Research* 28, no. 1 (2006): 97–103, https://doi.org/10.1179/016164106X91951.

2021 study looked at how acupuncture affected 30 people with vascular dementia, the second most common type of dementia after Alzheimer's disease. The participants received daily acupuncture treatments for 12 weeks. Researchers compared their blood work before and after the 12 weeks and found that not only did inflammation levels decrease by a whopping 20 percent, but their immune systems got stronger![223]

Acupuncture's immune-supporting effects could even help treat sepsis, an extreme response characterized by too much inflammation that often occurs in life-threatening infections.[224] Plus, there's substantial—and growing—evidence that acupuncture can reduce inflammation and even help reverse the organ damage that can happen as a result.[225]

FOREST BATHING

If I have to be in a research study, a walk in this one seems like a nice choice. Twenty healthy male university students were split into two groups: the city group and the forest group. Each group was driven to their assigned site, where they went on two guided hour-and-a-half walks. Then the groups went back to the same hotel, ate the same foods, and went to bed at the same time. The next day they were driven to a hospital to get lab tests done.[226]

---

223 Hui Zhi et al., "Acupuncture Can Regulate the Distribution of Lymphocyte Subsets and the Levels of Inflammatory Cytokines in Patients with Mild to Moderate Vascular Dementia," *Frontiers in Aging Neuroscience* 29 (November 29, 2021), https://doi.org/10.3389/fnagi.2021.747673.

224 Fang Lai et al., "Acupuncture at Zusanli (ST36) for Experimental Sepsis: A Systematic Review," *Evidence-Based Complementary and Alternative Medicine* 2020 (2020): 3620741, https://doi.org/10.1155/2020/3620741.

225 Ji-Eun Oh and Seung-Nam Kim, "Anti-Inflammatory Effects of Acupuncture at ST36 Point: A Literature Review in Animal Studies," *Frontiers in Immunology* 12 (January 11, 2022), https://doi.org/10.3389/fimmu.2021.813748; and Luis Ulloa, Salvador Quiroz-Gonzalez, and Rafael Torres-Rosas, "Nerve Stimulation: Immunomodulation and Control of Inflammation," *Trends in Molecular Medicine* 23, no. 12 (December 2017): 1103–120, https://doi.org/10.1016/j.molmed.2017.10.006.

226 Gen Xiang Mao et al., "Effects of Short-Term Forest Bathing on Human Health in a Broad-Leaved Evergreen Forest in Zhejiang Province, China," *Biomedical and Environmental Sciences* 25, no. 3 (2012): 317–24, http://dx.doi.org/10.3967/0895-3988.2012.03.010.

So: same length of walk, same food, same hotel. The only difference was "city" versus" forest." Would you expect there to be any difference in how their bodies reacted?

There were big differences, as it turned out. Compared to the city group, the forest group had lower oxidative stress, lower pro-inflammatory hormone levels, and less cortisol in their blood, *and* they reported a more positive mood.

And that's just, literally, a walk in the woods. Forest bathing goes beyond that.

Forest bathing isn't just about getting fresh air or being away from your screen, although those things can be beneficial. It involves paying particular, focused attention to the natural environment. It's basically a mindfulness practice like mindful eating or mindful breathing, but in a natural environment. A forest bathing session can be as short as half an hour in a city park. It could be part of an afternoon hike, or you could dive into it in more depth during an overnight trip.

Whatever approach you take, forest bathing can reduce stress hormones, improve sleep, reduce blood pressure, reduce the fight-or-flight nervous system state, and have a positive impact on levels of anxiety and depression.[227]

In part, that's because your mind has a powerful response to the natural world itself. As we saw earlier in the university student study, spending time in nature (as compared to in the city) can lower levels of stress and inflammatory blood markers.[228] Research shows that even just listening to natural sounds, rather than urban sounds, or looking at *pictures* of nature, can reduce stress.[229] Just having a

227 Qing Li, "Effects of Forest Environment (Shinrin-Yoku/Forest Bathing) on Health Promotion and Disease Prevention—The Establishment of 'Forest Medicine,'" *Environmental Health and Preventive Medicine* 27 (2022): 43, https://doi.org/10.1265/ehpm.22-00160.

228 Mao et al., "Effects of Short-Term Forest Bathing."

229 Cassandra D. Gould van Praag et al., "Mind-Wandering and Alterations to Default Mode Network Connectivity When Listening to Naturalistic Versus Artificial Sounds," *Scientific Reports* 7 (March 27, 2017): 45273, https://doi.org/10.1038/srep45273; and Daniel K. Brown, Jo L. Barton, and Valerie F. Gladwell, "Viewing Nature Scenes Positively Affects Recovery of Autonomic Function following Acute-Mental Stress," *Environmental Science & Technology* 47, no. 11 (June 4, 2013): 5562–69, https://doi.org/10.1021/es305019p.

hospital room with a window and natural light reduced the average length of stay in the intensive care unit at a hospital by 44 percent![230]

Oddly enough, virtual nature seems to have some of the same effects as "real" nature. A recent study showed that looking at virtual reality videos of nature reduced both anxiety and depression in college students.[231]

And medical professionals are taking notice. One Canadian program allows doctors to prescribe visits to Canada's national parks as a treatment for depression.[232] In the US, similar programs offer ways for doctors to make park visits more accessible to patients. Honestly, this blew me away when I heard about it. Doctors *prescribing* time in nature? That's big news.

What's even better is that natural environments can be a first step toward *preventing* some of these mental health issues in the first place. One study, for example, found higher levels of cognitive development and lower risk of emotional and behavioral problems when adolescents got more exposure to woodlands.[233]

Parents—take note!

Given that our bodies evolved in a natural environment, and we experience an unprecedented number of stressors in modern life, it's not surprising that combining mindfulness with time in nature can help you reduce stress and inflammation in a redwood-sized way.

230 Roxana Jafarifiroozabadi et al., "The Impact of Daylight and Window Views on Length of Stay among Patients with Heart Disease: A Retrospective Study in a Cardiac Intensive Care Unit," *Journal of Intensive Medicine* 3, no. 2 (April 2023): 155–64, https://doi.org/10.1016/j.jointm.2022.11.002.

231 Matthew H. E. M. Browning et al., "Daily Exposure to Virtual Nature Reduces Symptoms of Anxiety in College Students," *Scientific Reports* 13 (January 23, 2023): 1239, http://dx.doi.org/10.1038/s41598-023-28070-9.

232 Park Prescriptions, "PaRx: A Prescription Worth Filling," accessed May 12, 2023, https://www.parkprescriptions.ca/.

233 Mikaël J. A. Maes et al., "Benefit of Woodland and Other Natural Environments for Adolescents' Cognition and Mental Health," *Nature Sustainability* 4 (July 19, 2021): 851–58, https://www.nature.com/articles/s41893-021-00751-1.

TAI CHI

Although the practice of Tai Chi is likely more than 1,000 years old, it's inspiring brand-new science because of its impacts on mental and cognitive functioning. Tai Chi improves memory and executive function in people with mild cognitive impairment.[234] It improves inflammation and oxidative stress and reduces markers of neuroinflammation and neurodegenerative diseases. It improves neuroplasticity and is being studied for use in neurorehabilitation. It's an anti-inflammation, pro–mental health powerhouse.[235]

Tai Chi involves a set of slow, focused movements that activate the entire body and demand complete attention. The gentle movements, and the breathing and focus that go with them, combine the benefits of exercise with the DMN-deactivating properties of attention and focus.

In Chinese, Tai Chi means literally the "supreme ultimate." The name refers to the belief that Tai Chi brings together the two halves of the self and the cosmos: the yin and the yang, male and female, dark and light. Interestingly enough, one of its benefits is that it helps integrate the two halves, or hemispheres, of your brain. That's one reason it helps people with trauma.

You might mostly see old people doing it, but Tai Chi is an excellent practice for people of all ages, and getting started at any age is both rewarding and great for your health.

SENSORY DEPRIVATION

Ah, now *here's* the kind of mental health practice I can get behind.

Doing nothing.

---

234 Somporn Sungkarat et al., "Tai Chi Improves Cognition and Plasma BDNF in Older Adults with Mild Cognitive Impairment: A Randomized Controlled Trial," *Neurorehabilitation and Neural Repair* 32, no. 2 (February 2018): 142–49, https://doi.org/10.1177/1545968317753682.

235 Howe Liu and Yasser Salem, "Effects of Tai Chi on Biomarkers and Their Implication to Neurorehabilitation: A Systematic Review," *Innovation in Aging* 5, supplement 1 (2021): 895, https://doi.org/10.1093/geroni/igab046.3252.

Right? When you're stressed and tired and burnt out, what could possibly sound better than doing absolutely nothing?

Well, good news. Sensory deprivation is a specific way of doing nothing for an hour that can reduce anxiety and improve mood in people with stress-related conditions ranging from PTSD and panic disorder to generalized anxiety and social anxiety.[236] And that same form of "doing nothing" has demonstrated significant symptom reduction for anxiety disorders, as well as improvements in sleep, emotional regulation, and mood.[237]

I'd say that's some remarkable nothingness.

But why does sensory deprivation work? Every day, all day long, every second of the day, your body takes in sensory information and sends it to the brain. Touch. Sight. Sound. Smell. Taste. Even if you close your eyes, even if you are in the quietest room in your house, your senses are always gathering information.

Sensory deprivation lets all those information-gathering inputs just...take a break.

Most sensory deprivation involves what are known as float tanks. In a float tank, you float effortlessly in skin-temperature salt water in a closed, dark, quiet space. This reduction in stimulus provides a unique environment for your senses to quiet down and stop the constant flow of information. It allows you to feel comfortable and safe and helps switch your body out of stressed mode. More than that, it's a great experience.

Good News Fatigue

Historians tell us that civilization as we know it has been around for something like 6,000 years. Humans have been trying to find ways to

---

236 Justin S. Feinstein et al., "Examining the Short-Term Anxiolytic and Antidepressant Effect of Floatation-REST," *PLoS One* 13, no. 2 (February 2, 2018): e0190292, https://doi.org/10.1371/journal.pone.0190292.

237 Kristoffer Jonsson and Anette Kjellgren, "Promising Effects of Treatment with Flotation-REST (Restricted Environmental Stimulation Technique) As an Intervention for Generalized Anxiety Disorder (GAD): A Randomized Controlled Pilot Trial," *BMC Complementary Medicine and Therapies* 16 (March 25, 2016): 108, https://doi.org/10.1186/s12906-016-1089-x.

live longer, and better, and happier lives for that entire time—which explains why there are so many amazing practices to talk about in this chapter.

It's also why there's a chance you're getting "good news fatigue" right now.

Every one of the practices I'm talking about here? They're all good for fighting inflammation and reducing stress. As a result, it can feel like you've read the same thing over and over.

This fatigue break is just to remind you: you don't need to memorize the science behind these different methods, or remember which study relates to which one. Think of this chapter more like a menu.

What looks tasty? What might feel good or be easy to try? Where would you like to start?

The good news is that there are plenty of options! And you can come back and review the chapter anytime to get new ideas.

Now—back to our regularly scheduled chapter.

GARDENING

As a mental health practice, gardening might seem like it's a bit out of left field. (Ha ha, get it? Left *field*? Like in farming? Alrighty then.) But the science is in: gardening is healthy for you. Not only is it rewarding and satisfying to see the outcomes of your efforts and enjoy lots of happy plants in your life, but research shows that gardening has substantial mental and physical health benefits.

In 2015, a group of older women from a local community center in Seoul, South Korea, who gardened twice per week for eight weeks showed significant improvement in both their inflammation markers and their oxidative stress levels. Not only that, but their blood pressure stats improved, as did their cholesterol.[238]

---

238 Sin-Ae Park et al., "Gardening Intervention as a Low- to Moderate-Intensity Physical Activity for Improving Blood Lipid Profiles, Blood Pressure, Inflammation, and Oxidative Stress in Women over the Age of 70: A Pilot Study," *HortScience* 52, no. 1 (January 2017): 200–205, https://doi.org/10.21273/HORTSCI11232-16.

Even better, you don't even need to wait eight weeks to get the benefits of gardening. Gardening for just 20 minutes can have brain-health-boosting effects immediately. Researchers found that a brief gardening session increased their BDNF (see Chapter Five for a refresher), which has been shown to reverse age-related memory loss and improve cognitive function.[239]

Now that's what I'd call time well spent, even if you have to wait a while for your sunflowers to bloom.

What I love especially about gardening is how a broad range of people can get the benefits from it. While some practices might not be possible for those with mobility or cognitive challenges, gardening offers something for everyone. Gardening even improved cognition and daily living for a group of elderly people who were living in a high-care environment—people who weren't able to live on their own. They could still garden, and they still got the benefits from it, including improved cognition and improved ability to do their daily activities.[240]

So think about finding your green thumb. There are lots of great videos online that can help you get started.

GETTING HOT

Most of us love a hot bath every now and then. Sinking into the water can feel relaxing and rejuvenating, especially after a long day. But feeling better in the bath is about much more than just our muscles loosening up in the heat.

Used widely across Europe for thousands of years, thermal baths and saunas are now part of some healthcare systems, and they've

---

239 Sin-Ae Park et al., "Benefits of Gardening Activities for Cognitive Function According to Measurement of Brain Nerve Growth Factor Levels," *International Journal of Environmental Research and Public Health* 16, no. 5 (2019): 760, https://doi.org/10.3390/ijerph16050760.

240 Myong-Hwa Kim and Jung-Mi Kim, "The Effect of an Occupational Therapeutic Intervention Program Using Horticultural Therapy on Cognition and Daily Living Performance of the Elderly with Dementia," *Journal of Korean Society of Community-Based Occupational Therapy* 2, no. 1 (2012): 75–84, http://journal.kcbot.co.kr/sub/journal_detail.html?code=252070&?search=&year=2012&issueCode=18985.

been shown to provide benefits for people with a range of inflammatory conditions. A large-scale study conducted in Finland looked at the sauna habits of over 1,600 adults over 15 years. Researchers found that people who had four to seven sauna sessions per week substantially reduced their risk of strokes.[241] A similar study showed that frequent sauna sessions also lowered risks of dementia and Alzheimer's disease.[242]

It turns out that heating the body can have positive effects on the brain. In a study conducted at the University of Arizona, a group of participants who were diagnosed with clinical depression were "heated" up in a special device that increased their core body temperature to 101 degrees Fahrenheit. After a single session, the participants reported a substantial reduction in depressive symptoms that was apparent within one week of treatment and persisted through the six-week check-in.[243]

In another case, the same benefits were seen after the therapeutic application of warm mud.[244] Yeah, I know—being smeared in warm mud may not be your first choice. But the reduction in inflammation might well be worth it.

A more popular (and certainly drier!) way of getting hot quickly is to head to the sauna. Often associated with snowy climates, saunas aren't just a great way to escape the winter weather. Regular sauna use has a positive impact on system-wide inflammation. People using a sauna four to seven times a week had substantially reduced levels

241 Setor K. Kunutsor et al., "Sauna Bathing Reduces the Risk of Stroke in Finnish Men and Women: A Prospective Cohort Study," *Neurology* 90, no. 22 (May 29, 2018): e1937–44, https://doi.org/10.1212/WNL.0000000000005606.

242 Tanjaniina Laukkanen et al., "Sauna Bathing is Inversely Associated with Dementia and Alzheimer's Disease in Middle-Aged Finnish Men," *Age and Ageing* 46, no. 2 (March 2017): 245–49, https://doi.org/10.1093/ageing/afw212.

243 Clemens W. Janssen et al., "Whole-Body Hyperthermia for the Treatment of Major Depressive Disorder: A Randomized Clinical Trial," *JAMA Psychiatry* 73, no. 8 (August 2016): 789–95, https://doi.org/10.1001/jamapsychiatry.2016.1031.

244 Isabel Gálvez, Silvia Torres-Piles, and Eduardo Ortega-Rincón, "Balneotherapy, Immune System, and Stress Response: A Hormetic Strategy?," *International Journal of Molecular Sciences* 19, no. 6 (June 6, 2018): 1687, https://doi.org/10.3390/ijms19061687.

of C-reactive protein compared to people who only used it only once a week.[245]

And not to discourage movement, but one study that followed up with people after 11 years found that the reduction in inflammation from regular sauna use was comparable to that offered by regular exercise.[246] That's not to say that anything can replace movement (as we talked about in Chapter Five), but it's definitely a great addition.

GETTING COLD

Getting cold has become popular in the last decade in part because of the "Iceman," Wim Hof. He's best known for setting some icy world records, like longest distance swim under ice, climbing Mount Everest barefoot (!), and sitting submerged in a tank of ice water for over an hour. He's a pretty extreme example, but the basic idea behind what he does is supported by science: getting cold is good for your brain.

Research has shown that cold water immersion not only lowers heart rate, blood pressure, and cortisol levels, but also improves fatigue, pain, mood, and memory.[247]

Getting cold works in part because the shock focuses your mind without any effort on your part, essentially resetting the nervous system and bringing you into the present moment. Because your body can't tell the difference between a tiger, a stressful email, and the shock of cold water, regularly getting cold leads to a reduced stress and inflammatory response in general.[248] This is called cross-

---

245 Jari A. Laukkanen and Tanjaniina Laukkanen, "Sauna Bathing and Systemic Inflammation," *European Journal of Epidemiology* 33 (March 2018): 351–53, https://doi.org/10.1007/s10654-017-0335-y.

246 Setor K. Kunutsor, Tanjaniina Laukkanen, and Jari A. Laukkanen, "Longitudinal Associations of Sauna Bathing with Inflammation and Oxidative Stress: The KIHD Prospective Cohort Study," *Annals of Medicine* 50, no. 5 (2018): 437–42, https://doi.org/10.1080/07853890.2018.1489143.

247 A. Mooventhan and L. Nivethetha, "Scientific Evidence-Based Effects of Hydrotherapy on Various Systems of the Body," *North American Journal of Medical Sciences* 6, no. 5 (May 2014): 199–209, https://www.ncbi.nlm.nih.gov/pmc/articles/PMC4049052/.

248 M. J. Tipton, "Cold Water Immersion: Kill or Cure?," *Experimental Physiology* 102, no. 11 (November 1, 2017): 1335–55, https://doi.org/10.1113/EP086283.

adaptation. Your body gets used to the stress and dials down its response. It's a win–win.

But you don't have to go for midwinter runs in the Netherlands wearing nothing but underwear like the Iceman does.

The science on this is really new and very exciting. In a major breakthrough in 2015, scientists found that cold shock (and a special "cold shock protein" that is released) can actually create new synapses in your brain. Synapses are the connection points between neurons, and more synapses means better, faster, more efficient cognition. The study found that increasing the cold shock protein even has potential to protect against degenerative disorders like Alzheimer's. They also showed that the cold shock protein is lower in people with Alzheimer's disease.[249] Long story short: the more cold shock protein, the more protection for your brain.

These discoveries may lead to new ways to prevent and treat diseases like dementia.

Cold isn't just promising for long-term brain health though. In a study done on people who exercised, a group who reduced their core body temperature soon after exercising had less inflammation over the next few days.[250] And body cooling releases many of the same brain protection chemicals as are released during exercise.[251]

That's very cool. (Pun intended!)

I'll be coming back to temperature in Chapter Eleven, where we'll talk about new technologies that use cold to reduce inflammation and improve brain health. There is a lot of promise in these practices, but be aware that cold immersion can have its dangers if not done carefully. It's best to join a group or go to a clinic with experience in

---

249 Diego Peretti et al., "RBM3 Mediates Structural Plasticity and Protective Effects of Cooling in Neurodegeneration," *Nature* 518 (January 14, 2015): 236–39, https://doi.org/10.1038/nature14142.

250 Hervé Pournot et al., "Time-Course of Changes in Inflammatory Response after Whole-Body Cryotherapy Multi Exposures following Severe Exercise," *PLoS One* 6, no. 7 (July 28, 2011): e22748, https://doi.org/10.1371/journal.pone.0022748.

251 Diego Peretti et al., "TrkB Signaling Regulates the Cold-Shock Protein RBM3-Mediated Neuroprotection," *Life Science Alliance* 4, no. 4 (February 2021): e202000884, https://doi.org/10.26508/lsa.202000884.

cold immersion, at least at first. Or, if you want a gentle introduction, try just cooling your shower down a bit at a time.

It'll be worth it.

THE ISOLATION ISSUE

One of the benefits of all of these approaches is that, if you want to, you can do them with others. Even though most of them can be done on your own, even in your own home, getting together with other people turns out to be just as fundamentally important to your physical and mental health as the practices themselves.

People in Western countries are in the middle of what has been called a loneliness epidemic. Loneliness and lack of social interaction have been linked to chronic inflammation and poor physical and mental health, and with so many of us spending our time on our computers or at home, this isolation is only getting worse.[252]

Social interaction is a research-proven anti-inflammatory practice.[253] For some people, that's the world's best excuse to get all their friends together and celebrate. For others, especially introverts or shy people, it can be a bit harder. Fortunately, there are a lot of ways to meet your need for social connection.

Try getting together with a friend or family member for a meal once a week. Or get involved in a gardening club, volunteer group, or book club. Maybe you could get a friend involved in a new activity—or try

252 Karina Van Bogart et al., "The Association between Loneliness and Inflammation: Findings from an Older Adult Sample," *Frontiers in Behavioral Neuroscience* 15 (January 11, 2022), https://doi.org/10.3389/fnbeh.2021.801746.

253 Anna K. Forsman, Johanna Nordmyr, and Kristian Wahlbeck, "Psychosocial Interventions for the Promotion of Mental Health and the Prevention of Depression among Older Adults," *Health Promotion International* 26, supplement 1 (December 2011): i85–i107, https://doi.org/10.1093/heapro/dar074.

out one of the practices from this chapter. If you're not sure about how you'll get along with a particular group, you can sample a few classes until you find a teacher or a group you like and connect with.

Even just calling up a friend to chat can help your mental health and reduce stress and inflammation. It's not always easy to make connections, especially if you're dealing with mental health challenges, so take it one step at a time and focus on all the small wins along the way.

"IT SEEMS A LITTLE WEIRD, BUT IT'S WORKING"

When Jadyn's doctor first recommended that he try some new methods to reduce his stress, he was skeptical. He thought the doctor's ideas sounded weird. His aunt was into yoga, but other than that, he didn't know anyone who did things like floatation tanks. "Forest bathing" just sounded like an Instagram fad.

Not only did it sound strange, but he felt like he didn't have time. This was just another thing to add to his schedule when he was already feeling overwhelmed.

But his symptoms were really getting in the way of living his life, so he thought he might as well give it a try. He did not want to put off his search for a brand-new job another year, or even another month, if he could help it.

His first step was to find some yoga videos online. Feeling silly but willing to try anything, he put on his sweatpants and followed the first video in his living room. Some of the poses were hard, but to his surprise, he felt a little better afterward.

He also convinced a couple of friends to go with him to a local park. They even agreed to put their phones away for a few minutes and just look around. He didn't tell them he was "forest bathing" or doing mindfulness, but he did try out some of the stuff he'd read about. He focused his attention on a particular tree, then on his breathing.

At night, if he was feeling particularly stressed, he would put on a meditation app on his phone before bed. It turned out he slept better on the nights when he did that, and the following morning, he would wake up feeling more alert and more ready to think and work. He started using the short meditations every night.

His life wasn't transformed overnight, but pretty soon he felt consistently less stressed out. He was eating better and thinking more clearly. Over a couple of months of regular practice, he found himself starting to search job listings. Maybe he was ready to get out there and try again.

Jadyn's story is hopeful because, like a lot of people I've worked with, he found real benefits from the new practices he started. But taking on a new lifestyle change can be a big shift, especially for people who are living with mental health issues.

Sometimes, you need a jump start. A treatment that can be felt right away or after just a session or two. So that's where we're going next: cutting-edge treatments that can accelerate brain health in ways that, until recently, we didn't know were possible.

The anti-inflammation rocket boosters.

TL;DR

→ Alternative approaches are those you might do *instead of* Western methods like therapy or medication. Complementary approaches are those you might do *in addition*. I prefer complementary because you don't want to take any good options off the table.

→ The *default mode network* (DMN) is a system of brain areas that all fire together when you're not doing anything in particular—like if you're daydreaming. The *working memory network* (WMN) is a system of brain areas that fire together when you are actively working or thinking through something or engaged with an activity.

→ Too much time in the DMN has been linked to mental health issues like depression, anxiety, and PTSD. Complementary practices that engage your attention or pull your focus outside yourself can pull you out of the DMN.

→ There are many complementary practices you can engage with on your own, but don't let their simplicity fool you into thinking they can't have a powerful effect.

→ The wide range of complementary practices in this chapter, from forest bathing to cold plunging, have all been rigorously studied by scientists and shown to reduce chronic stress and inflammation—and improve mental health.

ACCELERATING BRAIN HEALTH

Cutting-Edge Approaches to Heal Your Brain

I know it's been a long road, but let me tell you, we're getting to the really exciting stuff now.

In Section Two, I introduced you to lifestyle changes that can reduce inflammation, improve mental health, and help your body and mind function at their best. But what if there were a way to get those benefits—to make those same functional changes in your mind and body—without the time and effort and resources required for lifestyle change?

Every single therapy, every approach, every practice in this book can move you toward better mental health. That doesn't mean they all work the same.

Think about planning a trip. There are lots of different ways to get to the same place. You can walk, ride a bike, drive, fly, take a train or a bus.

Let's say that optimal mental health is your destination. Lifestyle change is like walking there. It's predictable. It's steady. You don't need anyone else to help you do it. You could start right now. There are a lot of benefits—but it's not a fast way to get somewhere.

The guided practices in Section Three are like jumping on a plane. Sure, it's faster than walking, but you need an expert to fly it for you, it can be expensive, and you really want to make sure you're on a reputable airline. Plus, an airplane can't always get where you need to go. It can get you to the closest airport, but you still might need to walk or drive a ways. In your mental health journey, similarly, combining guided practices with lifestyle changes can make both more effective.

The technologies we'll cover in this section are totally different from the ones we've talked about before. They rely on the body's own processes, activating the kind of change that you would get from making consistent lifestyle changes. But they are much faster, getting you to your destination much faster than the months or years that lifestyle change usually requires.

ACCELERATING BRAIN HEALTH

Another way to think about these accelerators is like rocket boosters.

When a rocket launches, it needs thousands and thousands of tons of force to get it off the launchpad. It won't need anywhere near that much fuel later on, once it's already in flight. But the initial force of gravity is so strong that it needs rocket boosters to get it moving.

Bioaccelerators are the rocket boosters of this book. A *bioaccelerator* is any technology that activates natural systems and processes in your body, but provides the extra push that's needed to make progress quickly.

For example, while lifestyle changes like going to bed at the same time every night can dramatically improve your sleep over time, light and temperature technologies can tune into your brain's natural processes to improve sleep quickly and with much less effort. Similarly, a regular meditation practice can help quiet the default mode network over time, but psychedelics can achieve the same outcome almost completely, sometimes in a single session.[254]

Rocket boosters use the same fuel and provide the same upward motion as the regular engines on a rocket, but they contain so much *more* of it that they can push the heavy object faster, farther, and more easily upward.

The bioaccelerators in the next two chapters can do the same for your mental health, jump-starting or accelerating the effects of lifestyle changes, therapy, and other treatments.

HEALTHY BRAIN ACCELERATORS, NOT HACKS

Bioaccelerators aren't the same as biohacking. Biohacking refers to self-directed health enhancements. It's kind of like "DIY" for your

---

254 Haiteng Jiang et al., "Brain–Heart Interactions Underlying Traditional Tibetan Buddhist Meditation," *Cerebral Cortex* 30, no. 2 (February 2020): 439–50, https://doi.org/10.1093/cercor/bhz095; and Robin L. Carhart-Harris et al., "Neural Correlates of the Psychedelic State As Determined by fMRI Studies with Psilocybin," *Proceedings of the National Academy of Sciences USA* 109, no. 6 (January 23, 2012): 2138–43, https://doi.org/10.1073/pnas.1119598109.

body. Biohacking is generally popular with people who want to experiment with their bodies to push themselves to live longer or perform better. It can include everything from electronic "tattoos" (thin sensors that stick to your skin and gather data about you) to taking medications in off-label ways in the hope of creating certain changes in the body or brain.

There's nothing inherently wrong with biohacking or wanting to boost your performance or optimize your body. The problem with biohacking, especially from a mental health perspective, is that there's no clear definition about what it is. As a result, almost any practice, product, or method can use the biohacking label. I've seen people call surgically embedded headphones "biohacking," and I've also heard dieting referred to that way.[255] A lot of what people do to "hack" their bodies might be good, but a lot of it is experimental, untested, or not really a hack at all. A lot of biohacking methods push the boundaries of what's been studied and require expert-level knowledge to be used safely.

The technologies and approaches I'm going to talk about in this chapter are not about hacking. Hacking implies breaking in or doing something not quite legal, or safe, to get an outcome you want. We're not looking to break your body's source code. We want to amplify what's natural.

Bioaccelerators do just that. They accelerate or promote the optimal functioning of existing, natural body functions. Your body is already programmed to heal—bioaccelerators can help speed up that healing process.

Bioaccelerators amplify your body's natural ability to heal, to self-regulate, and to recover.

---

255 Caitlin Geng, "What to Know about Biohacking," Medical News Today, October 17, 2022, https://www.medicalnewstoday.com/articles/biohacking.

CHAPTER TEN

PSYCHEDELICS

From Forest and Festival to Breakthrough Therapy

Camilla has made substantial life changes and has found relief for the worst of her pain. She's sticking to her water aerobics, and there are days now when she has no pain at all.

But dealing with the physical symptoms has uncovered deeper concerns.

When she was in pain every day, Camilla didn't have the energy to address her long-standing self esteem and confidence issues. But now that the pain and exhaustion are under better control, she's started paying more attention to how her mental health is affecting her life in other ways. In particular, how it affects her relationships with her clients.

She first noticed the issue a few years ago when one of her new clients decided to work with a different therapist. It's a common occurrence in therapy. Sometimes a client and therapist just don't click.

The problem was, Camilla couldn't let it go. Her brain kept going over and over her meeting with the client. Nothing bad happened, but Camilla kept thinking about it. Why hadn't the client liked her?

She can tell herself a million times that she knows she's a good therapist. She is highly trained and highly regarded by her peers. Her patients give her positive feedback, and she can see them getting better.

Her inner critic doesn't seem to care about any of that. Every time, it still tells her she isn't as good as she should be. The thoughts and emotions are intrusive. She can't put them aside. They specifically bother her at bedtime when she's trying to relax, which makes it harder to sleep. Then she wakes up tired and doesn't feel prepared for work, setting the whole self-doubt cycle in motion again.

Now that the pain is under better control, she feels ready to tackle her anxiety and her self-esteem issues. She's had therapy herself, but this problem has proven very hard to budge. So she's intrigued when she reads about a new approach: psychedelic therapy. She asks her colleague, a well-respected psychiatrist, what he thinks. He says that he's seen psychedelics have great outcomes for people with issues like hers. Camilla is inspired to learn more, since he doesn't recommend anything without a sound scientific basis.

Camilla does her own research and decides to give it a try. It's a little bit scary, but the evidence is too strong to ignore.

MUCH MORE THAN PARTY DRUGS

It's hard to know exactly where to start when I talk to people about psychedelics. They can be phenomenal brain-health rocket boosters. The science is exciting and starting to really gain momentum. But they also have a bit of a reputation problem.

They're called treatments by some, mind expanding by others. Drugs. Party supplies. Healers.

So...which is it?

The short answer is, all of the above. The longer, more important answer, is that it depends a great deal on how, where, and why you use them.

There is a big difference between using these substances at home, or at a party, and using them in a therapeutic setting. When I talk about the brain health–boosting effects of psychedelics, I'm not talking about what happens in college dorms or at Burning Man.

I'm talking about medicine.

That's why this chapter is not so much about *psychedelics* as it is about *psychedelic therapy*.

Psychedelic therapy involves the medical management of a drug as a tool. The difference between someone using psychedelics on their own and psychedelic therapy is just like the difference between going to a physical therapy clinic and doing some shoulder exercises a friend told you about. In a therapy setting, the expert is an integral part of the process.

Psychedelics are potent compounds, and a trained therapist can tell you which ones to use, how to get the most out of them, and how to integrate and make sense of the experience.

But first things first. What exactly are psychedelics, anyway?

UNLOCKING NEW PERSPECTIVES

Psychedelics are part of a larger group of compounds referred to as *psychoactive*. A psychoactive compound (meaning it is "active on the psyche") is anything that alters or affects your state of mind.

Think about the difference between acetaminophen (Tylenol) and alcohol. Tylenol changes your body chemistry, but it doesn't change how you see things. It doesn't change how you perceive or understand the world. It just reduces pain. Alcohol, on the other hand, is psychoactive. It totally alters your perception. You might suddenly feel less inhibited or experience your surroundings differently. If you drink more, you may get confused or make different decisions than you normally would.

Psychoactive compounds can have all kinds of effects. They can be positive, harmful, or neutral. Even caffeine is mildly psychoactive, lifting mood and subtly shifting your mindset.

What all psychoactive compounds have in common is that they

interact with the nervous system to cause mood changes, behavior changes, or altered thoughts—or some combination of all of those.[256]

Psychedelics are a special category of psychoactive drugs.

Psychedelics shift the way you see yourself or the way you think about your own experiences. Rather than just lifting mood or giving you energy like caffeine, they can change your thinking.

As a result, psychedelics can help change long-standing mental patterns, including those associated with PTSD, depression, and anxiety.[257]

Some psychedelics are found in nature, while others have been created in labs. What they all have in common is that all psychedelic substances bind to the same group of receptors in the brain.

Binding to a receptor is like a key fitting into a lock.

Every cell in the human body is protected by a cell membrane. But cells can't be impenetrable. They need to let in food and chemical messengers and push out waste products. Receptors are the cell's way of determining what to let in and what to keep out.

Receptors are the doors in the membrane that open up into the cell. Each receptor recognizes a different shape of molecule. It's like a keyhole, and only the right chemical key will fit. Drugs and pharmaceuticals work because they bind to specific cell receptors—they're keys specially built for the cell's locks.

All psychedelics bind with the serotonin 5-hydroxytryptamine 2A (also known as 5-HT2A) group of receptors. That's why drugs like THC (the active compound in marijuana) aren't considered psyche-

256 Harris R. Lieberman et al., "The Effects of Caffeine and Aspirin on Mood and Performance," *Journal of Clinical Psychopharmacology* 7, no. 5 (October 1987): 315–20, https://journals.lww.com/psychopharmacology/abstract/1987/10000/the_effects_of_caffeine_and_aspirin_on_mood_and.4.aspx.

257 Jennifer M. Mitchell et al., "MDMA-Assisted Therapy for Severe PTSD: A Randomized, Double-Blind, Placebo-Controlled Phase 3 Study," *Nature Medicine* 27 (May 10, 2021): 1025–33, https://www.nature.com/articles/s41591-021-01336-3; Guy M. Goodwin et al., "Single-Dose Psilocybin for a Treatment-Resistant Episode of Major Depression," *New England Journal of Medicine* 387 (November 3, 2022): 1637–48, https://doi.org/10.1056/nejmoa2206443; and Joseph M. Rootman et al., "Adults Who Microdose Psychedelics Report Health Related Motivations and Lower Levels of Anxiety and Depression Compared to Non-Microdosers," *Scientific Reports* 11 (November 18, 2021): 22479, https://doi.org/10.1038/s41598-021-01811-4.

delics, even though they are psychoactive. They don't bind to that receptor group.

The other thing all psychedelics have in common is their deactivating effect on the DMN. Remember our discussion about the default mode network, the group of brain areas that get activated when we're not thinking about anything in particular? Remember how spending too much time in the DMN is strongly correlated with depression, anxiety, PTSD, and other mental health issues?

Psychedelics act as rocket boosters in large part because they help us rapidly quiet the DMN and "reboot" the brain.

Specifically, we call psychedelics bioaccelerators because they both mimic and massively accelerate the effects of other practices that quiet the DMN but might take years or even decades to work.

One incredible example is the veteran with PTSD whose DMN activity shifted so much after *one single session* of MDMA therapy that it looked exactly like the DMN of an expert meditator who'd logged thousands of hours meditating.[258]

That is bioacceleration at its best: tapping into the body's natural ability to heal itself and kicking it into high gear.

We'll come back to the different types of psychedelics and the research that supports their use. But first, let's get at the deeper question: Why do these drugs work?

REBOOT YOUR BRAIN

Psychedelics work because they help us break old patterns and create new ones.

In Chapter Nine, you learned about some ways to break out of DMN activation. What psychedelics do is similar, except for the magnitude of impact.

---

258 S. Parker Singleton et al., "Altered Brain Activity and Functional Connectivity after MDMA-Assisted Therapy for Post-Traumatic Stress Disorder," *Frontiers in Psychiatry* 13 (January 11, 2023), https://doi.org/10.3389/fpsyt.2022.947622.

While activities like yoga and cold plunging can engage your brain and quiet the DMN over time, psychedelics can totally rewrite your old patterns really quickly. Sometimes even in a single session. And they make it easier to build new patterns to replace them.

Psychedelics are a shortcut. Psychedelics not only quiet the DMN, but they reduce the energy needed to create new patterns. They can even stimulate the growth of new neurons, generating all-new pathways in your brain.[259]

Old thought patterns are like sledding tracks. When you're out sledding, if the hill is smooth and the snow is fresh, you can go any way you want. But if there is already a deep groove where people have sledded over and over, you can get stuck in that groove, and then it's hard to go in any other direction.

People with a diagnosis of obsessive-compulsive disorder (OCD), for example, have brains that respond too much to errors and not enough to their brain's "it's okay to move on from this" signals. So they stay stuck in check-and-correct loops, checking the stove or washing their hands over and over again.[260]

Something similar happens to all of us, whether we have a mental health diagnosis or not.

When we're in our normal patterns, we reinforce the same old connections over and over, and they become rigid. Some connections get used all the time, while others tend to lie dormant. The connections you use a lot get more and more ingrained, while the ones you use less often become harder to access or are even forgotten.

As the neuropsychologist Donald Hebb put it, "Neurons that fire together, wire together."[261] In other words, if two parts of the brain

259 Cato M. H. de Vos, Natasha L. Mason, and Kim P. C. Kuypers, "Psychedelics and Neuroplasticity: A Systematic Review Unraveling the Biological Underpinnings of Psychedelics," *Frontiers in Psychiatry* 12 (September 9, 2021), https://doi.org/10.3389/fpsyt.2021.724606.

260 Luke J. Norman et al., "Error Processing and Inhibitory Control in Obsessive-Compulsive Disorder: A Meta-Analysis Using Statistical Parametric Maps," *Biological Psychiatry* 85, no. 9 (May 1, 2019): 713–25, https://doi.org/10.1016/j.biopsych.2018.11.010.

261 "How Neurons That Wire Together Fire Together," Neuroscience.com, December 23, 2021, https://neurosciencenews.com/wire-fire-neurons-19835/.

work at the same time, they get reinforced. The pathways between them become faster and more automatic. The more your brain repeats a pattern, the more ingrained it becomes.

Psychedelic therapy is like starting over again with a clean surface. It's like there was a big snowstorm overnight, and all the old sledding paths have been filled in. It's all fresh again. That allows you to step outside of the neural pathways you normally use. Not only does it immediately break you out of the painful thought cycles, but it gives you the space and energy to create new ones. Better, healthier ones.

New studies have revealed that psychedelics also create more communication all around the brain. Different parts of the brain that don't normally talk to each other suddenly connect. This allows new connections to be formed between parts that don't normally speak to each other.[262]

And that's not just theory. These new patterns have been shown to shift everything from addiction and anxiety to depression and PTSD.[263]

THE THREE Ns

As if all that weren't enough, psychedelics also increase *neuroplasticity, neurogenesis, and neuroprotection.*

For a long time, scientists thought that the brain became fixed and stopped changing as soon as you reached adulthood. They basically

262 S. Parker Singleton et al., "Receptor-Informed Network Control Theory Links LSD and Psilocybin to a Flattening of the Brain's Control Energy Landscape," *Nature Communications* 13 (October 3, 2022): 5812, https://doi.org/10.1038/s41467-022-33578-1.

263 Pim B. van der Meer et al., "Therapeutic Effect of Psilocybin in Addiction: A Systematic Review," *Frontiers in Psychiatry* 14 (February 8, 2023), https://doi.org/10.3389/fpsyt.2023.1134454; Neil M. Weston et al., "Historic Psychedelic Drug Trials and the Treatment of Anxiety Disorders," *Depression & Anxiety* 37, no. 12 (December 2020): 1261–79, https://doi.org/10.1002/da.23065; R. L. Carhart-Harris et al., "Psilocybin with Psychological Support for Treatment-Resistant Depression: Six-Month Follow-Up," *Psychopharmacology* 235 (2018): 399–408, https://doi.org/10.1007/s00213-017-4771-x; and Tracey Varker et al., "Efficacy of Psychoactive Drugs for the Treatment of Posttraumatic Stress Disorder: A Systematic Review of MDMA, Ketamine, LSD and Psilocybin," *Journal of Psychoactive Drugs* 53, no. 1 (2021): 85–95, https://doi.org/10.1080/02791072.2020.1817639.

thought that once you reached your mid-20s your brain (and mind) were sealed in plaster and never changed again.

Nothing could be further from the truth.

The brain is constantly remapping itself. Learning creates new physical connections among neurons all the time. When people lose their vision or hearing through disease or injury, their brains remap the "vision" or "hearing" areas of the brain to do other work.[264] That's *incredible.*

Forget anything you've ever heard about "only using 10 percent of your brain." The truth is the exact opposite: the brain doesn't allow a single neuron to go to waste.

Your brain's ability to reorganize itself is called *neuroplasticity,* and it's unbelievable news for people with hard-to-treat mental health issues. It means that even the most stubborn brain pathways, like those associated with OCD, can be shifted. You're not stuck with the cognitive patterns you learned as a child or the brain pathways dug by your depression.

Psychedelics also stimulate *neurogenesis.*[265] That means growing new neurons. Until very recently, it was believed that the brain was basically the only part of your body that never grew new cells and couldn't be repaired. Not true! Very recent science shows that new cell growth can continue in at least some parts of the brain throughout your life. New neurons means even more new connections and new opportunities to think and act and feel differently. New neurons contain new potential for a healthy mind.

The icing on the cake is that psychedelics also appear to be *neuroprotective.*[266] That's just what it sounds like: protecting your brain's cells from damage. Psychedelics can increase individual neurons' resil-

---

264 Gabriella V. Hirsch, Corinna M. Bauer, and Lotfi B. Merabet, "Using Structural and Functional Brain Imaging to Uncover How the Brain Adapts to Blindness," *Journal of Psychiatry and Brain Functions* 2, no. 7 (2015), http://dx.doi.org/10.7243/2055-3447-2-7.

265 De Vos, Mason, and Kuypers, "Psychedelics and Neuroplasticity."

266 Shariq Mansoor Khan et al., "Psychedelics for Brain Injury: A Mini-Review," *Frontiers in Neurology* 12 (July 28, 2021), https://doi.org/10.3389/fneur.2021.685085.

ience. Remember when we talked about being stuck in the stress cycle and how stressors can cause physical damage to the brain? Psychedelics heal existing damage, sure, but their neuroprotective effects mean they can help make your brain less susceptible to *future* damage too.

What might seem even more surprising is that psychedelics can help protect against physical damage to the brain. Recent studies suggest that psychedelic therapy may help heal the effects of traumatic brain injuries like concussions, rebuilding brain cells and reshaping the existing healthy cells to take on activities from the injured areas. In other words, psychedelics don't just affect the mind in an abstract way—they promote repair and resilience in the physical brain itself.

THE INFLAMMATION CONNECTION

In addition to facilitating changes in neural patterns, psychedelics also appear to directly block inflammation.

I mentioned that all psychedelics bind to the same type of receptors in the brain. That's what they all have in common. What new studies are showing is that activating this particular receptor group has powerful anti-inflammatory effects.

There's a reason I call psychedelic therapy a brain-health accelerator! But you don't have to just take my word for it. The FDA thinks so too.

THE WAR ON (THERAPEUTIC) DRUGS

Before we talk about the studies that are now proving the value of psychedelics for mental health, we need to take a little detour. When I tell people how exciting these substances are and about their mind-blowing potential to change how we treat depression, anxiety, and other mental health problems, they often ask me the same question: *How come we didn't know this before?*

The fact is, research on psychedelics started in the 1960s and even earlier. (And of course, indigenous societies knew about their benefits much earlier, even if they didn't study them scientifically.) But just as scientists were starting to make progress in understanding psychedelics, the War on Drugs put a stop to their work.

At the time, because there wasn't a lot of understanding about psychedelics, they were lumped in with all the other illicit drugs. Anything that had ever been used or sold as a "street," or recreational, drug was lumped together as potentially dangerous. As a result, almost no research could be done on psychedelics for decades.[267]

BREAKTHROUGH STATUS

FDA approval is one of the most important steps in getting a medication into the hands of people who need it.

Up until about the 1980s, the FDA reviewed every new drug using the same tried-and-true process. Every drug had to go through multiple, large studies and meet very strict guidelines for acceptance. And every drug, whether it was for runny noses or for cancer, was evaluated on a first-come, first-served basis.

The problem was, the review process could take years—and patients weren't having it. They wanted the FDA to prioritize certain drugs. If a new drug was designed to treat a condition that didn't have any treatments yet, or if it had the potential to be a lot better than what was currently available, patients thought the FDA should put it first in line.

Eventually, the FDA agreed. They changed their rules to meet patients' demands. One of those new rules, put into law in 2012, was the Breakthrough Therapy designation.

The FDA defines a Breakthrough Therapy as one with the promise to treat a serious condition better than any existing therapy already on the market.[268] In other words, to get a Breakthrough Therapy

---

267 Joshua Falcon, "Situating Psychedelics and the War on Drugs within the Decolonization of Consciousness," *ACME* 20, no. 2 (2021): 151–70, https://acme-journal.org/index.php/acme/article/view/1947.

268 U.S. Food & Drug Administration, "Breakthrough Therapy," For Patients, January 4, 2018, https://www.fda.gov/patients/fast-track-breakthrough-therapy-accelerated-approval-priority-review/breakthrough-therapy.

designation, a new drug or treatment can't just show potential. It can't just be pretty good. There has to be evidence suggesting it's substantially better than anything that's available now.

Some psychedelics have already started earning this special status.

In 2017, the FDA granted MDMA (sometimes known as "ecstasy") breakthrough status for treating PTSD. And then in 2019, they designated psilocybin (the active ingredient in so-called magic mushrooms) as a breakthrough drug for major depressive disorder.

Both PTSD and major depressive disorder already have treatments on the market. Giving psychedelics Breakthrough Therapy designations shows that the FDA thinks psychedelics have the potential to be significantly better than any of the already-available drugs for treating these conditions.

The designation matters, not only because it shows the potential of psychedelics, but because it can speed up the research. New treatments with Breakthrough Therapy designation get reviewed by the FDA faster. Researchers are allowed to work more directly with the FDA throughout the study process. And getting a Breakthrough Therapy designation can convince more researchers to study that substance.

So far, only one psychedelic, ketamine, has full FDA approval. It was approved in 2019 for treatment-resistant depression.

But there are a lot more potential approvals in the works. The data are starting to come in from early studies of a wide variety of psychedelics, and the results are *stunning*. I'm going to introduce you to the most promising of them all, starting with the depression-fighting powerhouse once known as Special K.

KETAMINE

Ketamine is an anesthetic—in other words, it's a strong painkiller and sedative. It's like the anesthesia you were under if you got your wisdom teeth removed, but the difference between ketamine and other types of anesthesia is that ketamine works really quickly and doesn't slow your heart rate (which is often what makes "going under anesthesia" dangerous when you're having a surgical procedure).[269]

The FDA approved ketamine as a general anesthetic in 1970.[270] It was used by American soldiers during the Vietnam War for battlefield surgery, but it wasn't until 2000 that researchers at Yale School of Medicine published the first clinical study to show ketamine's antidepressant effects. That study found that a *single dose* of ketamine improved depression significantly—sometimes even helping patients to a near-complete recovery.

The truly amazing part was that this recovery occurred in less than 24 hours. It took *one day* to resolve cases of depression that, for some participants, had been plaguing them for years. And the dose they were given was less than what would even be needed for anesthesia.[271]

No wonder the researchers described their findings as "robust." Seems like a bit of an understatement.

Ketamine has also shown surprising promise in treating alcohol use disorder. Like PTSD, alcohol use disorder is very difficult to treat. Most drugs are ineffective, and therapy often doesn't work. That's why it was breaking news when a study published in 2022 reported that six months after treatment with ketamine, 86 percent of the study participants were still abstinent from alcohol. And the mortality rate for these patients declined 90 percent in the year following the study, compared to those not treated.[272]

---

269 Paolo Vincenzi et al., "Continuous Thoracic Spinal Anesthesia with Local Anesthetic Plus Midazolam and Ketamine Is Superior to Local Anesthetic Plus Fentanyl in Major Abdominal Surgery," *Surgery Open Science* 2, no. 4 (October 2020): 5–11, https://doi.org/10.1016/j.sopen.2020.07.002; and S. J. Barker, D. M. Gamel, and K. K. Tremper, "Cardiovascular Effects of Anesthesia and Operation," *Critical Care Clinics* 3, no. 2 (April 1987): 251–68, https://pubmed.ncbi.nlm.nih.gov/3332199/.

270 Parke Davis, "Ketamine Hydrochloride (Ketalar)," *Clinical Pharmacology & Therapeutics* 11, no. 5 (September 1970): 777–80, https://doi.org/10.1002/cpt197011 5777.

271 Robert M. Berman et al., "Antidepressant Effects of Ketamine in Depressed Patients," *Biological Psychiatry* 47, no. 4 (February 15, 2000): 351–54, https://doi.org/10.1016/S0006-3223(99)00230-9.

272 Meryem Grabski et al., "Adjunctive Ketamine with Relapse Prevention–Based Psychological Therapy in the Treatment of Alcohol Use Disorder," *American Journal of Psychiatry* 197, no. 2 (February 2022): 152–62, https://doi.org/10.1176/appi.ajp.2021.21030277.

For such a difficult and complex condition, that is a staggering result.

And you want to know what's even more staggering? For the first time in history, the FDA has approved a psychedelic as medicine.

It's a ketamine-based nasal spray, approved to treat depression (alongside an oral antidepressant). And it's specially approved for people whose depression hasn't responded to other treatments. So people with chronic, long-lasting, hard-to-treat depression.

Which makes it absolutely crazy that, in the study that led to the FDA approval, the patients saw substantial improvement in as little as *two days*.[273]

Until recently, that kind of improvement was considered absolutely impossible for people with treatment-resistant depression. Psychedelics are finally moving the needle for folks like these, and it's about time!

PSILOCYBIN

Psilocybin (pronounced *sill-oh-sigh-bin*) is what Camilla chose to start with in her psychedelic therapy.

When her doctor first recommended it, all she could think was, *Wait, isn't that what's in "magic mushrooms"?* She was concerned. She'd heard weird stories about things happening to people who took these kinds of mushrooms at concerts or festivals.

And yeah, psilocybin has been used by some people as a so-called party drug. But it turns out psilocybin can also be a powerful tool in the mental health toolbox.

Psilocybin is a naturally occurring compound found in more than 200 species of fungi. It's been used by cultures all over the world for thousands of years, and now, finally, it's being studied as well.

---

273 US Food & Drug Administration, "FDA Approves New Nasal Spray Medication for Treatment-Resistant Depression; Available Only at a Certified Doctor's Office or Clinic," press release, March 5, 2019, https://www.fda.gov/news-events/press-announcements/fda-approves-new-nasal-spray-medication-treatment-resistant-depression-available-only-certified.

In fact, psilocybin is the focus of the biggest study of psychedelics for mental health that's ever been done.

The Compass Pathways trial uses a combination of psilocybin and talk therapy for treatment-resistant depression. Like with ketamine, these are patients whose depression is chronic, life-altering, and not responding to existing therapies.

The early-released results show that some of the patients getting psilocybin showed no signs of depression *at all* 12 weeks later—twice as many as in the group that didn't get psilocybin.

Psilocybin appears to be a light at the end of a very dark tunnel for many people with depression that just hasn't gotten better with any other treatment.

LSD

Almost everyone has heard of *lysergic acid diethylamide*, or LSD. What most people don't know is that it was discovered by accident.

In 1938, a Swiss chemist named Albert Hofmann was trying to create a new stimulant drug. He ended up with LSD instead.

In fact, Hofmann didn't even recognize the potential of his new discovery until later. He put aside the LSD compound at first and didn't discover its psychedelic properties until he tested it on himself five years later! (I would certainly never recommend that someone "try out" a new chemical on themselves—but there were fewer rules about that kind of thing in the 1930s.)

When Hofmann tried LSD himself, he found that it totally altered his perception of himself and his surroundings. It affected his mood and made him see everyday things very differently. He continued to experiment with it, and over time, other scientists and psychiatrists began to experiment with it as well. Although it hadn't been tested in any clinical trials yet, psychiatrists believed it might change patients' perceptions of themselves and help them achieve new insights into their lives.

Even the US Army got involved, experimenting with LSD to find out whether it could be used as a mind-control drug.[274] Rest assured, though: it didn't work. LSD changes your perception, but it can't be used to control you. Thanks to cultural backlash, LSD was put aside and not studied for decades. Now, finally, scientists are looking at it again.

In a recent, groundbreaking Phase II clinical trial, researchers investigated the potential of LSD combined with psychotherapy for treating anxiety disorders. The study recruited 42 participants, half of whom also had life-threatening illnesses like cancer.

The results were striking. Patients who received LSD experienced *11 times greater* reductions in anxiety compared to those given a placebo. Not only that, but the study revealed that the effects lasted up to 16 weeks—*and* the patients in the LSD group also showed improvements in secondary outcomes such as depression and OCD. This research really highlights the promising prospects of psychedelic treatments, shedding light on a novel approach to managing anxiety and related disorders.[275]

DMT

DMT (full name *N,N-Dimethyltryptamine*) is a compound that is naturally produced in our brains and can also be synthesized and ingested. It's also the active part of ayahuasca, a brew made by traditional cultures in South America. Weirdly, the brain appears to suddenly release a large volume of DMT during a near-death experience, and it's thought that DMT may play a role in dreams and imagination.

In fact, a DMT session can sometimes feel like a near-death expe-

274 Terry Gross, "The CIA's Secret Quest for Mind Control: Torture, LSD and a 'Poisoner in Chief,'" *NPR*, September 9, 2019, https://www.npr.org/2019/09/09/758989641/the-cias-secret-quest-for-mind-control-torture-lsd-and-a-poisoner-in-chief.

275 Friederike Holze et al., "Lysergic Acid Diethylamide–Assisted Therapy in Patients with Anxiety with and without a Life-Threatening Illness: A Randomized, Double-Blind, Placebo-Controlled Phase II Study," *Biological Psychiatry* 93, no. 3 (February 1, 2023): 215–23, https://pubmed.ncbi.nlm.nih.gov/36266118/.

rience. A group of researchers compared reports from near-death experiences to the reports of healthy people who took DMT. The people who took DMT reported almost exactly the same experiences as the people who had near-death experiences. They gave remarkably similar descriptions of what they saw and reported a similar increase in their ability to get fully immersed in their environment and in the present moment.[276] Most of these experiences were positive and life-affirming, and not frightening.

There's not enough research yet to know what role DMT plays in near-death experiences, but the similarities do show us how powerful a DMT session can be.[277]

One 2022 study found that people using ayahuasca for the first time saw a substantial reduction in depression and other symptoms after just one session. More than 80 percent of them still showed improvement in their symptoms when the researchers followed up six months later.[278]

But remember what I said about being "powerful enough to help, powerful enough to hurt"? It applies especially to these psychedelics. They've gotten a popular reputation through social media, adventure travel, and people calling themselves "shamans," but there's no regulation for these activities, and psychedelics can be as dangerous as any strong medicine.

Though perception changes in the last decade have resulted in ayahuasca ceremonies being seen as a safe and generally positive life experience, the research demonstrates that using DMT or ayahuasca in a nonclinical study could result in persistent psychological issues (in as much as 20 percent of regular users), and participants

276 Christopher Timmermann et al., "DMT Models the Near-Death Experience," *Frontiers in Psychology* 9 (August 14, 2018), https://doi.org/10.3389/fpsyg.2018.01424.

277 Charlotte Martial et al., "Neurochemical Models of Near-Death Experiences: A Large-Scale Study Based on the Semantic Similarity of Written Reports," *Consciousness and Cognition* 69 (March 2019): 52–69, https://doi.org/10.1016/j.concog.2019.01.011.

278 Daniel F. Jiménez-Garrido et al., "Effects of Ayahuasca on Mental Health and Quality of Life in Naïve Users: A Longitudinal and Cross-Sectional Study Combination," *Scientific Reports* 10 (March 5, 2020): 4075, https://doi.org/10.1038/s41598-020-61169-x.

with previous mental health challenges are more likely to experience negative effects.[279] Significantly, in a nonclinical setting there is no consideration for your context and history, and no medical supervision during or importantly after the experience.

MDMA

Candy. Dancing shoes. Disco biscuits. *Scooby Snacks?*

A.k.a., ecstasy.

Despite a negative reputation (from its use on the party and rave scene), MDMA has shown a great deal of potential in helping people with anxiety and PTSD. Because of its effect on mood and its ability to increase empathy and sensations of pleasure, MDMA can help people who struggle with negative emotions and memories.

MDMA has a lot of names. As a street or party drug, it's often called *ecstasy* because a sense of happiness or euphoria is one of its most common effects. Part of the reason for the nicknames is that the real name of MDMA is so long most people never bother to use it, even those who study it. Technically, it's called *Methylenedioxy methamphetamine.* (See why nobody bothers with that name?)

For anyone thinking its recreational use makes it safe to try for mental health reasons, it's worth noting that these days, most party drugs are laced with fentanyl, a deadly anesthetic. Medical and therapeutic uses in clinics and labs use only pure forms of MDMA.

In 2021, the Multidisciplinary Association for Psychedelic Studies (MAPS) released the results of a trial using MDMA to treat severe PTSD.[280] The MAPS trial is the first-ever Phase III clinical trial for *any* psychedelic. That's important because Phase III is the final stage usually required for FDA approval. It means that the drug has already

---

279 Rebecka Bremler et al., "Case Analysis of Long-Term Negative Psychological Responses to Psychedelics." *Scientific Reports* 13 (September 25, 2023): 15998, https://doi.org/10.1038/s41598-023-41145-x.

280 Mitchell et al., "MDMA-Assisted Therapy for Severe PTSD."

been determined to be safe and is now being tested to find out if it effectively treats patients with a specific condition.

The results have been *incredible*. More than two-thirds of the patients who were treated with MDMA no longer qualified for a PTSD diagnosis after just three sessions.[281]

This is so mind blowing it bears repeating. After just three sessions, these patients, some of whom struggled with PTSD for decades, were no longer considered to even *have* PTSD. No existing therapy comes close to being this effective, much less this effective this quickly.

BREAKING SCIENCE

Up until now, the "psychedelic experience" part of psychedelics has been considered a core, or at least an inevitable, part of the treatment. It was assumed that in order to get the benefits, you had to experience the feelings, thoughts, visions, or other mind-altering aspects of psychedelics. That might be changing.

The US military's research division was recently awarded $27 million to develop compounds with the same therapeutic effects as psychedelics, without the "trip" or hallucinations. Last year, the group announced that they had succeeded. They'd created a compound that hits the same brain receptor as psychedelics and provides just as much of an antidepressant effect (at least in mice), but without the psychedelic experience.[282]

The effect hasn't yet been studied in humans, but for those who are not sure about the subjective experience of psychedelics but want the benefits, this is exciting news.

---

281 Mitchell et al., "MDMA-Assisted Therapy for Severe PTSD."

282 UNC School of Medicine Pharmacology, "Scientists Create Non-Psychedelic Compound with Same Anti-Depressant Effect," Faculty News, October 14, 2022, https://www.med.unc.edu/pharm/scientists-create-non-psychedelic-compound-with-same-anti-depressant-effect/.

If you want to know more about what the experience of each of these psychedelics is like, check out Michael Pollan's book *How to Change Your Mind*. He describes many of them in great detail.

But keep in mind—he didn't take these substances in a therapeutic context. If you are using them to work through difficult material or treat mental health issues, it's best to seek out an expert to help you.

PSYCHEDELICS AS THERAPY

Psychedelic therapy is not the same as taking psychedelics at a concert or at a party. Like any other form of professional therapy, it's done with a trained expert in a controlled setting.

In this context, psychedelics are tools with the potential to help you make progress faster. They can essentially speed up the process of therapy, which could otherwise take months or years.

In other words, psychedelics don't necessarily replace therapy, but they can definitely accelerate it.

For example, when people who were trying to quit smoking combined psilocybin with CBT, they had a lot more success than people who did CBT only.[283]

Like any kind of therapy, different approaches will look different. Depending on what substance is involved and what methodology the therapist uses, a psychedelic therapy session can take anywhere from an hour to six hours or sometimes more. Some sessions might be guided like talk therapy, encouraging you to actively work through issues. Other sessions allow you to just experience the psychedelic's effects and then discuss your insights afterward.

What they all have in common is that there is a trained clinical expert present. And in every case, the expert's job is to help you work through, understand, and integrate the experience.

---

283 Matthew W. Johnson, Albert Garcia-Romeu, and Roland R. Griffiths, "Long-Term Follow-Up of Psilocybin-Facilitated Smoking Cessation," *American Journal of Drug and Alcohol Abuse* 43, no. 1 (2017): 55–60, https://doi.org/10.3109/00952990.2016.1170135.

WHAT TO EXPECT

Although the types of therapy and the specifics of the sessions look different, all professional, effective psychedelic therapies should share three elements in common: preparation, experience, and integration.

Preparation

The first step of any professional psychedelic therapy session is preparation. Psychedelics can change your perception of yourself. They can rewire your brain and break old mental patterns. These experiences can change your life for the better in so many ways—but they are also totally new to most of us. Going straight into a psychedelic experience with no preparation can be a setup for not getting what you need out of it, or for having a difficult or stressful experience.

Any trained therapist working with psychedelics should provide enough preparation to make you feel comfortable with what's going to happen. They should explain what substance you will be taking, how many sessions are involved, and how long the sessions should last. They will likely also help you understand your goals for the session and what the experience will be like.

The most important element of preparation, though, is talking with your therapist about your background and issues and what medications or therapies you are already using. Health history, substance use problems, mental health status, and medications can change the way you experience everything in your life, and that includes psychedelics. Use of SSRIs, for example, can dampen the effects of certain psychedelics and create potential toxic effects when combined with others.[284]

---

284 Collin M. Price, Allison A. Feduccia, and Katrina DeBonis, "Effects of Selective Serotonin Reuptake Inhibitor Use on 3,4-Methylenedioxymethamphetamine-Assisted Therapy for Posttraumatic Stress Disorder: A Review of the Evidence, Neurological Plausibility, and Clinical Significance," *Journal of Clinical Psychopharmacology* 42, no. 5 (September/October 2022): 464–69, https://doi.org/10.1097/jcp.0000000000001595; and Simon Ruffell et al., "The Pharmacological Interaction of Compounds in Ayahuasca: A Systematic Review," *Brazilian Journal of Psychiatry* 42, no. 6 (November–December 2020): 646–56, https://doi.org/10.1590/1516-4446-2020-0884.

If you walk into a "clinic" and are offered a psychedelic session without a trained clinician, with no preparation, or without providing a complete medical and psychological history, you should consider going elsewhere.

Like any therapy, the success of a psychedelic session depends on how you approach it, how comfortable and safe you feel in it, and how well trained your clinician is. Seek out clinical professionals with background and training in psychedelics and in your specific issues.

Session

The second step is the session itself. Whenever you and your therapist decide you are ready, you will set up a time, go to the clinic or your therapist's office, discuss what is going to happen, and then ingest or receive an injection of the substance.

You may have someone monitoring your vital signs during the session. Your session might be active, with your therapist talking you through the experience. MDMA sessions for PTSD, for example, often involve talking about your traumatic experiences while you're using the MDMA. Other substances, like psilocybin, are more passive. In those sessions, you will simply experience whatever comes up, although you are likely to have a medical monitor in the room with you to monitor your progress and discuss what's happening if necessary.

Integration

Finally, the third phase is called integration. I know I've mentioned this already, but in case you missed it, psychedelics are *powerful drugs*. Remember our motto: "If it's powerful enough to help, it's powerful enough to hurt." Anything that can change your brain is going to have a profound effect on you. That's why talking through and understanding your experience is so important.

Integration is an opportunity to talk about, understand, and make sense of your psychedelic experience. It's also when you will start to actively apply your psychedelic insights to your mental health challenges.

In a sense, psychedelics prime your system. They help clear out the debris and open you up to new ways of thinking and being. But they can't create brand-new patterns on their own. Developing new patterns, and understanding how your old patterns have been showing up in your life, depends on what you do following the session.

The integration phase may include one session, or it might require a longer course of therapy. Exactly what integration will look like depends on your goals for psychedelic therapy and the underlying issues you are dealing with. The key is that integrating the experience allows you to understand it and use it to create new thoughts and behaviors in your life.

RECOMMENDATIONS

What I said before about pharmaceuticals and supplements is even more true for psychedelics. Because these substances can have an enormous impact on your mental health, you need to be careful how you use them.

WORK WITH AN EXPERT IN A CONTROLLED, CLINICAL SETTING

There are a lot of reasons to work with a trained therapist or clinician when you're trying psychedelic therapy. We already mentioned some of the considerations to take into account before deciding whether this type of therapy is right for you, such as your medical history and possible interactions with other medications.

Another potential risk is that without the proper care and preparation, some psychedelic experiences can lead to re-traumatization. If you have a significant trauma history or are currently experiencing a mental health crisis, you might decide you don't want to start psychedelic therapy quite yet. You and your therapist should talk about how to get stable before deciding whether this option works for you.

CONSIDER THE LEGALITY OF THE SUBSTANCE AND HOW YOU WILL ACCESS IT

Currently, the only federally legal psychedelic treatment in the US is ketamine. In other countries, legality and prescribing of substances varies. For example, Canada has legalized the ability for doctors to prescribe psychedelic therapy. This is a double-edged sword. On one hand, ketamine is easier to access than some of the other psychedelics (some of which you can only get if you participate in a clinical trial). On the other hand, quite a few ketamine clinics have opened up to take advantage of its legality, and not all of them employ professionals who are trained in this form of therapy.

That's why it's critical that you do your research before you choose a clinic.

Look for providers who clearly consider what they're doing to be therapeutic. They should consider psychedelic therapy a medical treatment, and their clinic should look like a medical facility, not a day spa or yoga studio. Any expert psychedelic therapy will include comprehensive pretreatment counseling and posttreatment support. There should be medical staff on site.

If they let you walk in and take a psychedelic right away, you should walk out!

CONSIDER BEING PART OF A CLINICAL TRIAL

Although some people are afraid to be in a psychedelic clinical trial, the benefits can be great. You get top-notch care, no matter what treatment you are getting. You are monitored more often, and often by higher-trained clinical staff, than if you went to a regular clinic. Plus, you can get access to extremely promising drugs that could help you more than what's on the market now.

That said, getting involved in a clinical trial isn't for everyone, and it's not always possible to access one even if you'd like to. If this is an avenue you are considering, take a look at the MAPS website (maps.org) or the AIMS Institute (aimsinstitute.net) to find out more.

DEFEATING OLD PATTERNS

After Camilla's first psilocybin-assisted therapy session, she felt pretty raw, like she'd been through weeks of therapy in a single day. The clinician she worked with warned her about this, so she'd already arranged to take a couple days off work. That meant she was able to go home and sleep a lot, then spend the next day taking things slowly.

The morning after that, she saw her first client since the psychedelic experience, and she noticed that her mood was very different. She was hopeful and positive, even though this client had been difficult in the past. Throughout the day, she found herself being less reactive. If something happened that she didn't expect, she didn't immediately get stressed and worried.

Best of all, her constant self-criticism seemed to be backing off. When one of her long-time clients decided to end therapy, she didn't spend days wondering what she did wrong. Now, she doesn't toss and turn at night, wondering if she even deserves to be a therapist or if she'll ever get another client. And her personal relationships feel deeper because she's not constantly worried about whether the other person will reject her.

Challenging sessions with clients, and challenging situations with friends or family, don't push her over the edge or hit her as hard as they used to.

Even though she's a therapist, she never realized how much her childhood experiences were affecting her life. The underlying emotional challenges have been with her so long, it's like they became invisible. Like that was just "who she was." Now she's seeing that it doesn't have to be. Thoughts and behaviors she's lived with for decades are starting to have less of a hold on her.

Not everyone benefits from psychedelic therapy as much as Camilla did. As a therapist herself, Camilla had years of experience with the process of therapy, and she was able to find an experienced professional to work with. Not everyone has that starting foundation to draw from.

But the new science about psychedelics is extremely promising. These substances are showing benefits far beyond SSRIs, and beyond talk therapy alone, across a wide spectrum of mental health conditions and symptoms.

If psychedelics aren't for you, though, or if you want to try a different kind of brain-health accelerator, take heart. Not all cutting-edge treatments have to go into your body. And not all of them involve medicines or talking.

Some of the most encouraging and hopeful research is looking at how to use new technologies to directly affect the brain itself. That's where bioacceleration really takes off.

TL;DR

→ *Bioaccelerators* are tools that turn on, power up, or otherwise increase your body's own ability to repair.

→ Psychedelics are *bioaccelerating compounds* that change how you perceive the world and yourself. They provide new perspectives and can both rewire your brain and physically heal it.

→ Psychedelics have been scientifically demonstrated to be effective in reducing inflammation and dramatically improving mental health, sometimes in just a single session.

→ Psychedelic therapy (also known as psychedelic-assisted therapy) is not the same thing as taking psychedelics on your own or at a festival. Psychedelic therapy integrates the experience into a process that involves preparation ahead of time and integration (making sense of it) afterward. Always look for a reputable, trained therapist.

→ Despite very promising research results, not all psychedelics are legal everywhere. If you're interested in trying it, look for a medical clinic that offers legitimate psychedelic therapy.

CHAPTER ELEVEN

———

BIOACCELERATING WITH BRAIN HEALTH TECHNOLOGIES

For the first time today, Ash is able to close the door to their office, sit down for a minute, and relax. It's tax time, and everything is go-go-go all day. Everyone in the office is busy, but Ash is especially overwhelmed. After years of hard work, they finally got their promotion—just in time for a major new client to switch to an entirely new accounting system two months before their taxes were due.

Ash can handle it. This is their specialty. It's why they got the promotion. But it's also a lot. Ash has moments when they wonder if they are working more than is reasonable.

Without quite thinking about it, Ash fills their coffee mug again from the espresso machine in their office and settles down at their computer. Since they have a minute, they decide to pull up the stress and health data on their smart watch and...it is not great.

Their stress score is way up. Ash digs deeper, scanning the numbers from the last few days.

Heart rate: elevated most of the time and wildly erratic during a particularly tense two-hour meeting earlier this morning.

Walking steps: almost none today, almost none yesterday, almost none the day before that.

And the sleep data doesn't look great, either, which bothers Ash a lot. When things were slower, they were able to get their sleep habits under control, and it made a big difference in their stress level. But now, with everyone in the office at maximum capacity and tax day creeping closer every minute, Ash is overloaded. Even with all their new lifestyle changes—eating better, taking the vitamins their doctor recommended, going through their sleep routine every night—their system can't keep up.

The balance has shifted. Before, even though there was stress, there was also enough downtime to allow Ash's self-care routines to work. Now, the stress is too high and too constant to be handled with the changes Ash has already made. They feel like they've tipped over into the red zone, revving their engine without going anywhere, putting wear and tear on their body all the time, even just sitting here.

Glancing once more at the data on their screen, Ash realizes that as long as the stress keeps piling on, what they're already doing isn't going to be enough. They need something powerful to tip the system back into balance.

HOUSTON, WE HAVE LIFT-OFF

You know the old phrase, "Save the best for last"?

Well, I don't want to say that we've saved the best for last, exactly. Every single method, approach, and recommendation in this book has the potential to fight inflammation, improve your mental health, and radically improve your quality of life.

That said…we've saved some of the most exciting, most rocket-boosting, most potentially life-improving interventions for this final chapter.

Whether you're like Ash and you've tried a lot of other methods and gotten benefits but are still struggling with symptoms, or if you want to jump-start your inflammation-fighting plan right from the get-go, these potent bioaccelerators can help.

That's why we call these the true rocket boosters of mental health.

TECHNOLOGIES FOR WELLNESS

Every human culture has used whatever technology it had available to treat disease—even when that "technology" was just a sharpened stone. The very earliest modern humans used splints to help set broken bones, and in the past 50 years, medical devices like pacemakers, cochlear implants, and implanted glucose monitors have made it obvious that new technologies can play an even more critical role in human health.

And it's a good thing because modern life has its own set of new challenges. We sit too much. We're indoors too much. We get too much artificial or computer-screen light and not enough natural light. We're stressed and constantly bombarded with stimuli. All of these modern stressors can take away from our ability to achieve optimal well-being.

A lot of the newer health technologies are designed to make up for those challenges. These are the brain-health accelerators, facilitating the same kinds of brain changes that Ash made with their sleep routine, only faster.

Some people who try these technologies feel better after a *single session*. That's what bioacceleration looks like.

The technologies that work best are those that accelerate or speed up natural processes in your body. They don't work against your body or fight it. Instead, they amp up your body's own natural healing and recovery.

You could get a lot of the same benefits by totally changing your diet, sleep patterns, physical activity, and lifestyle. For many of us, given the responsibilities and realities of our lives, these kinds of changes feel close to impossible.

The technologies in this chapter can provide the same kinds of brain-health benefits, inflammation-fighting power, and symptom improvement in days or weeks, without having to revamp your entire life.

RATE OF REPAIR

When I bought my 40-year-old house, I remember being ecstatic. No more landlord! No more upstairs neighbors blasting music at 2:00 a.m.!

I had been in the house less than two months when a surprise wind storm blew down a tree on my property—right onto my deck. That's when I realized that no landlord also meant no one to call when something broke. I did some research, found a deck guy online, paid a heartbreaking amount of money to fix the gaping hole, and went on with my life.

A month later, it was termites. Six months later, the refrigerator and the washing machine died within a week of each other.

Two years in, the roof needed to be replaced—and while the roof guys were up there working, they discovered a hole in the attic siding that had to be patched.

You get the idea. Owning a home is a privilege, but it's also an exercise in constant maintenance. There's always something broken, something that should be replaced soon, something that's making a weird noise you should probably get looked at…

No house will ever reach a state of home-owning nirvana where everything works and stays working forever.

As long as it's a small repair here and one new appliance there, you can manage it. The disaster happens when too many repairs are needed all at once, and you don't have the time, money, or energy to deal with all of them. This often happens with older homes in particular. If nothing has been maintained or replaced for a long time, everything starts to fall apart at the same time, and it becomes harder and harder to keep up.

Your body is like that too.

Your body experiences damage every single day, whether it's

something obvious like a cut on your finger or more subtle like the damage caused by polluted air. Fortunately, you also have natural repair processes that keep working all the time to keep up.

When your overall function is high—when you are doing well generally—your repair systems can keep up with the damage. But sometimes the repairs fall behind, or the damage occurs too quickly for your body to keep up. You reach a threshold where stressors overwhelm the functioning of your repair systems.

That overwhelm is experienced as symptoms. The further your body is pushed beyond that threshold, the worse the symptoms get. The rate of damage is faster than the rate of repair.

When that happens, you need help to push your body back into balance.

Even worse, your body's repair systems might actually slow down as your symptoms get worse—and your rate of repair slows down naturally as you age. So every year, your repair systems work a little slower, but you keep adding new damage.

The technologies in this chapter are accelerators for your rate of repair.

SAY HELLO TO THE ACCELERATORS

The thing about an accelerator is that it has to, you know, *accelerate* something. So what is it, exactly, that bioaccelerators...accelerate?

As you go about your day, there are two main influences on how you feel: what's going on outside yourself, and what's going on inside. Bioaccelerator technologies can work on either of these. Some of them boost positive influences from the external environment, while others reset or shift your internal environment.

The two types of accelerators work a bit differently. Like supplements, the external environment accelerators generally concentrate something that's good for you. For example, your body naturally responds positively to certain kinds of light, so concentrating your exposure to those kinds of light can power up your recovery.

The internal environment accelerators tend to work a bit differently. Instead of concentrating something outside yourself, they reset an internal system, something that's already happening inside you. For example, training your brain waves into new patterns can substantially relieve stress and allow your body and mind to heal.

All of them kick your body's own natural healing and balancing mechanisms into high gear.

EXTERNAL ACCELERATORS

Picture it: the dawn of life on Earth. Single-celled organisms float around in a soup of nutrients, absorbing and dividing and generally taking it easy. They are basking in the luck of winning the one-in-a-million lottery of being on a planet with all the right conditions for life to start up at all.

A lot of pieces had to come together to make Earth habitable: the right mix of chemicals, the right temperature. But two things in particular supported early life forms: sunlight and oxygen.

In the billions of years since then, a lot has changed. We have legs and use ATMs and play Angry Birds. What hasn't changed is that our bodies need—and respond to—sunlight and oxygen. No matter how technologically advanced we get, our bodies are still evolved from those earliest life forms. Certain wavelengths of light can shift our moods, even our cognitive abilities, and can help overcome the negative effects of lack of sleep.[285] Getting more oxygen to our cells promotes healing and pushes us toward health.[286]

The difficulty is that we don't live in the primordial soup anymore.

---

285 T. A. Bedrosian and R. J. Nelson, "Timing of Light Exposure Affects Mood and Brain Circuits," *Translational Psychiatry* 7 (January 31, 2017): e1017, https://doi.org/10.1038/tp.2016.262; Sarah Laxhmi Chellappa et al., "Non-Visual Effects of Light on Melatonin, Alertness and Cognitive Performance: Can Blue-Enriched Light Keep Us Alert?," *PLoS ONE* 6, no. 1 (January 26, 2011): e16429, https://doi.org/10.1371/journal.pone.0016429; and Leilah K. Grant et al., "Daytime Exposure to Short Wavelength-Enriched Light Improves Cognitive Performance in Sleep-Restricted College-Age Adults," *Frontiers in Neurology* 12 (February 21, 2021), https://doi.org/10.3389/fneur.2021.624217.

286 Paul Trayhurn, "Oxygen—A Critical, But Overlooked, Nutrient," *Frontiers in Nutrition* 6 (February 12, 2019), https://doi.org/10.3389/fnut.2019.00010.

We can't just float around absorbing what we need. Making up the difference is what external accelerators are for.

Reset with Light Therapies

Just to show how important light is, let's talk about darkness for a second.

Experiments studying how people respond to total darkness have discovered some strange and, frankly, disturbing outcomes.

When people live in total darkness for days or weeks at a time, they start to lose their internal clocks. They have no idea how much time has passed, when they should sleep and wake up, or what time it is outside. Their bodies react with chaos, not getting enough sleep or sleeping too much, not knowing when to eat, not digesting effectively.[287]

Even weirder, being in a dimly lit room makes people more likely to lie or act selfishly.[288] Long periods without enough light make doctors and nurses more likely to make dangerous or even fatal mistakes with medication.[289] People who live and work in places that don't get a lot of light (like inside the Arctic Circle) or work night shifts are more likely to get certain kinds of cancer and chronic illnesses.[290]

Kids who sit in darker corners of a classroom do worse on tests than kids sitting near windows.[291]

287 J. N. Mills, D. S. Minors, and J. M. Waterhouse, "The Circadian Rhythms of Human Subjects without Timepieces or Indication of the Alternation of Day and Night," *Journal of Physiology* 240, no. 3 (August 1, 1974): 567–94, https://doi.org/10.1113/jphysiol.1974.sp010623.

288 Wen-Bin Chiou and Ying-Yao Cheng, "In Broad Daylight, We Trust in God! Brightness, the Salience of Morality, and Ethical Behavior," *Journal of Environmental Psychology* 36 (December 2013): 37–42, https://doi.org/10.1016/j.jenvp.2013.07.005.

289 C. Roseman and J. M. Booker, "Workload and Environmental Factors in Hospital Medication Errors," *Nursing Research* 44, no. 4 (July–August 1995): 226–30, https://pubmed.ncbi.nlm.nih.gov/7624233/.

290 X-S. Wang et al., "Shift Work and Chronic Disease: The Epidemiological Evidence," *Occupational Medicine* 61, no. 2 (March 1, 2011): 78–89, https://doi.org/10.1093/occmed/kqr001.

291 Lisa Heschong, Roger L. Wright, and Stacia Okura, "Daylighting Impacts on Human Performance in School," *Journal of the Illuminating Engineering Society* 31, no. 2 (2002): 101–114, https://doi.org/10.108 0/00994480.2002.10748396.

(I literally just went and opened the blinds after reading through that research again. Even I have to be reminded about how important these things are.)

The thing is, not all light is created equal, as far as our health is concerned. Different types and intensities of light activate different processes in the body. Morning light tends to stimulate your body, while evening light tells it to start winding down for rest.

Scientists have even identified specific wavelengths of light that have specific effects on the body. The process is called *photobiomodulation*. Light ("photo") affects your body ("bio"), changing it ("modulating" it) throughout the day. So photobiomodulation refers to how different types of light have different effects on your body and mind.

Exposing yourself to different frequencies or intensities of light can help your body and mind reset in their natural patterns, encouraging healing and promoting ideal sleep and waking cycles.

Let's look at a couple of popular, and well-supported, types of light therapy.

Red Light Therapy

Remember that old commercial for dish soap that said, "Softens hands while you do dishes"?

Well, red light therapy was discovered because scientists working with plants found that the lights they were using actually *healed their hands* when they worked under them.

They were using red light because it helps plants with photosynthesis. But the more they worked with the plants, the more they saw cuts and scrapes on their hands healing faster.

That research was funded by NASA, so the researchers automatically wondered how red lights might be useful in space. Being in space can cause muscles to become weak from lack of resistance, and wounds don't heal very well either. So when they saw the effects of red light on their own hands, the plant scientists started to think, *Could this be used by astronauts?*[292]

The answer was yes—and that was the beginning of medical uses of light therapy.

Red light refers to frequencies of light that are near the infrared end of the spectrum. In humans, it's active on the skin, rather than through the eyes. So most red light therapies involve skin exposure, often using nothing more complicated than a red-light lamp.

Red light therapy is now recommended for not only skin conditions (which you might expect), but also for a range of brain and mental health disorders including depression, traumatic brain injury, stroke, Parkinson's disease, and Alzheimer's disease.[293] It's a simple intervention with potentially profound effects.

Light Therapy

Light therapy is intentional exposure to the kind of light we usually get outside in the morning or in the summertime.

There's a reason we often feel happier during the summer, and it's not just being on vacation. The light is actually different. Because of the earth's relationship to the sun during different seasons, the light in summer is brighter. In the winter, the sun is lower in the sky, meaning the light is more indirect. You're not getting as much benefit.[294] Plus, all of us tend to hunker down inside during the winter, meaning you're less likely to get sun at all.

The best thing about light therapy is that sessions as little as 30 minutes at a time can increase job satisfaction, reduce stress, and

---

292 NASA Spinoff, "NASA Research Illuminates Medical Uses of Light," NASA Technology Transfer Program, May 19, 2022, https://spinoff.nasa.gov/NASA-Research-Illuminates-Medical-Uses-of-Light.

293 Michael R. Hamblin, "Shining Light on the Head: Photobiomodulation for Brain Disorders," *BBA Clinical* 6 (December 2016): 113–24, https://doi.org/10.1016/j.bbacli.2016.09.002.

294 Shia T. Kent et al., "Effect of Sunlight Exposure on Cognitive Function among Depressed and Non-Depressed Participants: A REGARDS Cross-Sectional Study," *Environmental Health* 8 (July 28, 2009): 34, https://doi.org/10.1186%2F1476-069X-8-34.

improve symptoms of depression, anxiety, and fatigue.[295] People with seasonal affective disorder (SAD) were found to have reduced their depression after a *single* one-hour session.[296]

Plus, it's super accessible, with light-therapy lamps available for home use or in clinics and some spas.

THE LIGHT FANTASTIC: NEW RESEARCH IN LIGHT THERAPY

In case all that isn't enough, new studies are demonstrating the power of light therapy all the time, even in conditions and diseases that have historically been hard to treat.

Brain Injury and TBIs: It makes sense that light affects wake and sleep cycles, energy levels, and even focus and concentration. But light therapy for physical brain injuries? The science is starting to say yes. One 2016 study, for example, exposed mice to red light twice a day before a brain injury. After the injury, the mice who'd been exposed to light recovered more of their cognitive and physical functions within 24 hours and had lower inflammation levels than the mice without light exposure. Red light exposure *protected* their brains against the worst effects of a physical injury.[297]

295 Mihyang An et al., "Why We Need More Nature at Work: Effects of Natural Elements and Sunlight on Employee Mental Health and Work Attitudes," *PLoS ONE* 11, no. 5 (2016): e0155614, https://doi.org/10.1371/journal.pone.0155614; and Julia Maruani and Pierre Alexis Geoffroy, "Bright Light as a Personalized Precision Treatment of Mood Disorders," *Frontiers in Psychiatry* 10 (February 28, 2019), https://doi.org/10.3389/fpsyt.2019.00085.

296 Gloria M. Reeves et al., "Improvement in Depression Scores after 1 Hour of Light Therapy in Patients with Seasonal Affective Disorder," *Journal of Nervous and Mental Disease* 200, no. 1 (January 2012): 51–55, https://doi.org/10.1097/nmd.0b013e31823e56ca.

297 Hae In Lee et al., "Pre-Conditioning with Transcranial Low-Level Light Therapy Reduces Neuroinflammation and Protects Blood-Brain Barrier after Focal Cerebral Ischemia in Mice," *Restorative Neurology and Neuroscience* 34, no. 2 (March 21, 2016): 201–214, https://doi.org/10.3233/rnn-150559.

And it's not just mice who benefit. Another study in 2022 found that veterans with histories of TBI (traumatic brain injury) who got 60 minutes of bright light therapy every morning for four weeks saw dramatic reductions in their symptoms. Their concussion severity scores went down by 16 percent, measures of poor sleep symptoms reduced by 23 percent, and scores indicating negative mood decreased by 27 percent.[298]

Alzheimer's and Parkinson's: Research is also showing benefits from light therapy for people living with Alzheimer's and Parkinson's, devastating conditions with very few effective therapies. Researchers in 2019 showed that Alzheimer's and Parkinson's patients treated with light therapy improved in their executive skills, recall, and task switching, among other positive outcomes.[299] And another 2017 study of red light therapy in Parkinson's patients showed that sleep quality improved by 21 percent, daytime sleepiness dropped by 29 percent, and physical activity went up by 18 percent.[300]

That's some impressive accelerating power.

None of these light technologies are expensive or super high tech. They are effective specifically because they aren't strange or new. They make use of the natural processes already at work in your brain and body.

You could say you evolved to respond to them.

---

298 Jonathan E. Elliott et al., "Feasibility and Preliminary Efficacy for Morning Bright Light Therapy to Improve Sleep and Plasma Markers in US Veterans with TBI. A Prospective, Open-Label, Single-Arm Trial," *PLoS ONE* 17, no. 4 (April 14, 2022): e0262955, https://doi.org/10.1371/journal.pone.0262955.

299 Marvin H. Berman and Trent W. Nichols, "Treatment of Neurodegeneration: Integrating Photobiomodulation and Neurofeedback in Alzheimer's Dementia and Parkinson's: A Review," *Photobiomodulation, Photomedicine, and Laser Surgery* 37, no. 10 (October 2019): 623–34, https://doi.org/10.1089/photob.2019.4685.

300 Aleksandar Videnovic et al., "Timed Light Therapy for Sleep and Daytime Sleepiness Associated with Parkinson Disease: A Randomized Clinical Trial," *JAMA Neurology* 74, no. 4 (2017): 411–18, https://doi.org/10.1001/jamaneurol.2016.5192.

In addition to light, your body also needs oxygen to survive and thrive.

Although—step back a second. We talk about the body like it's one thing: a single unit that acts and heals and responds as a whole. But every single cell is also its own smaller unit, acting on its own, living and healing and dying in its own time.

Every single cell is its own little power factory. It takes in oxygen and food and converts them into energy to make your heart pump, your fingernails grow, your neurons fire, and all the other activities that are going on in your body all the time.

What that means is that every single individual cell in your body needs oxygen to thrive. It's not enough just to get oxygen into your body. It needs to be able to reach each cell—just like we talked about in Chapter Five.

There are all kinds of reasons why your cells might be starved for oxygen or not getting enough. A sedentary lifestyle is one. Inflammation is another. Whatever the reason, the outcome is the same. Decreased oxygen to the limbs or extremities (fingers and toes) can cause numbness or tissue damage.[301] Decreased oxygen to the brain can cause all kinds of symptoms, from anxiety and brain fog to depression and fatigue.

COVID-19 was, unfortunately, a reminder of how important oxygen is to the brain. Low oxygen in COVID-19 patients caused all kinds of havoc, from inflammation and tissue damage to persistent brain fog.[302]

Remember, your brain uses 20 percent of your total oxygen intake. So limited oxygen can affect it the most. That's why external acceler-

---

301 R. M. Leach and D. F. Treacher, "Oxygen Transport2. Tissue Hypoxia," *BMJ* 317 (November 14, 1998): 1370, https://doi.org/10.1136/bmj.317.7169.1370.

302 Leif Østergaard, "SARS CoV-2 Related Microvascular Damage and Symptoms during and after COVID-19: Consequences of Capillary Transit-Time Changes, Tissue Hypoxia and Inflammation," *Physiological Reports* 9, no. 3 (February 2021): e14726, https://doi.org/10.14814/phy2.14726; and Damilola D. Adingupu et al., "Brain Hypoxia, Neurocognitive Impairment, and Quality of Life in People Post-COVID-19," *Journal of Neurology* 270 (2023): 3303–314, https://doi.org/10.1007/s00415-023-11767-2.

ators that help you get more oxygen to your cells promote all kinds of positive outcomes.

Hyperbaric Chambers

One form of oxygen therapy you might have heard of is called a *hyperbaric chamber*. These chambers are most commonly used for recovery from decompression sickness in scuba divers—also known as "the bends." When divers come up too quickly, the pressure around their bodies decreases, and air bubbles get trapped in the blood. These bubbles can cause symptoms from joint pain to death.

The hyperbaric chamber creates a pressurized environment, reducing the bubbles in the blood and making oxygen more available to cells.

But hyperbaric chambers aren't just for the bends. Researchers have found that they reduce neuroinflammation in a variety of conditions including brain injury, stroke, and even long COVID-19.[303]

Hyperbaric chambers used to be extremely rare, but now most hospitals have them, and some wellness centers even offer hyperbaric oxygen therapy.

Exercise with Oxygen Therapy (EWOT)

Exercise with oxygen therapy is just what it sounds like: exercising while breathing concentrated oxygen. Like a hyperbaric chamber, exercise with oxygen therapy saturates your cells with oxygen so that it gets to all the small vessels throughout your body. Only instead of lying down in a large pressurized chamber, you wear a mask that delivers oxygen into your body while you increase your heart rate.

---

303 Guanghui Xiu et al., "Role of Hyperbaric Oxygen Therapy in PDGF-BB-Mediated Astrogliosis in Traumatic Brain Injury Rats Associated with ERK 1/2 Signaling Pathway Inhibition," *European Journal of Medical Research* 28 (February 25, 2023): 99, https://doi.org/10.1186/s40001-023-01062-1; Wei-Wei Zhai et al., "Hyperbaric Oxygen Therapy in Experimental and Clinical Stroke," *Medical Gas Research* 6, no. 2 (April–June 2016): 111–18, https://doi.org/10.4103/2045-9912.184721; and Aisha M. Bhaiyat et al., "Hyperbaric Oxygen Treatment for Long Coronavirus Disease-19: A Case Report," *Journal of Medical Case Reports* 16 (February 15, 2022): 80, https://doi.org/10.1186%2Fs13256-022-03287-w.

The combination of increasing your heart rate and getting more concentrated oxygen means the oxygen is more easily dissolved into the bloodstream and becomes more easily available to your cells. Various forms of concentrated oxygen and exercise with oxygen therapy have been shown to fight inflammation, reduce symptoms like stress and anxiety, and even reduce the risk of strokes and cancer.[304]

But guess what? The opposite can, paradoxically, also sometimes be true.

Wait a Minute—*Less* Oxygen Can Be Good?

It makes sense that *concentrated* oxygen would be good for you. But wouldn't you assume that restricting oxygen would have the opposite effect?

Not always.

A 2019 Nobel Prize–winning medical team discovered that oxygen restriction, or *hypoxia*, can actually lead to positive health outcomes.

Hypoxia is a state in which your cells don't get enough oxygen to maintain homeostasis. Your body always wants to stay in balance, so when something is off, your body immediately tries to set it right. When you get too hot, you sweat to cool yourself off. When you get too cold, you shiver to warm yourself up. Similarly, when your cells don't get enough oxygen, your body fights back by increasing its neuroprotective responses.

The effects tend to be positive and anti-inflammatory. Responding to low blood oxygen can actually stimulate your body to grow new blood vessels to get more oxygen to your cells, and in at least some cases, they can stimulate the growth of new brain cells as well.[305]

---

304 Mark Sircus, *Anti-Inflammatory Oxygen Therapy: Your Complete Guide to Understanding and Using Natural Oxygen Therapy* (New York: Square One Publishers, 2015).

305 Takuya Hashimoto and Futoshi Shibasaki, "Hypoxia-Inducible Factor as an Angiogenic Master Switch," *Frontiers in Pediatrics* 3 (April 24, 2015), https://doi.org/10.3389/fped.2015.00033; and Debia Wakhloo et al., "Functional Hypoxia Drives Neuroplasticity and Neurogenesis via Brain Erythropoietin," *Nature Communications* 11 (March 9, 2020): 1313, https://doi.org/10.1038/s41467-020-15041-1.

The science on this is very new and extremely complicated, and there's still debate about why and how the benefits might occur.

What is clear is that sometimes, not getting enough oxygen to your cells can be *good* for you. These findings could help explain part of why intense exercise is beneficial. If you exercise hard enough to make cells hypoxic, even briefly, your body releases the chemicals to get you back in balance—with positive results.

In fact, elite athletes have been using this trick for ages. I went to college in Flagstaff, Arizona, which is at about 7,000 feet. That's a very high altitude, meaning there's less oxygen in the air. When I went swimming at the university swimming pool, I'd see the Japanese Olympic swimming team working out in the lane next to me! They wanted that low-oxygen, high-altitude training benefit.

What is worth remembering is that *selective, intentional* stress on your system (like exercise) can trigger your body into healing mode. However, stress can only be beneficial if your body can handle it.

INTERNAL ACCELERATORS

As we've evolved, humans have developed complex systems to keep ourselves safe and thriving. Instead of relying on the external environment to provide what we need, we have an entire ecosystem inside ourselves. We carry around our own life-support package. So even though we still rely on external inputs like sunlight and oxygen, we also have our own internal environment to rely on.

The accelerators in this section are directed at that internal environment. Rather than providing a concentrated dose of something external, they boost or shift something that's already inside you.

Regulate Your Hormones

Letting your arm fall asleep is rarely something you do on purpose. But it turns out that *intentionally* restricting blood flow can increase strength gains in athletes, improve memory and cognition in older adults, and improve the symptoms of multiple sclerosis (MS).[306]

What happens when you restrict blood flow has a lot to do with hormones.

We've talked about hormones before, so I'm not going to go into a lot of detail here. Short version: hormones are chemical messengers, turning on and off various processes in your body.

One of the major players in your optimal functioning is called human growth hormone, or HGH. HGH is used by your body for a ton of different purposes, from digestion and metabolism to neuroprotection.[307] It might seem like something called "growth hormone" would only be important for kids, but that's not the case. HGH controls or influences dozens of systems in the body throughout your life. HGH is so important that some diseases are now treated directly with HGH injections.[308]

Blood flow restriction (BFR) turns out to be an HGH bioaccelerator.

Origins of Blood Flow Restriction

BFR can be traced back to a single person: Yoshiaki Sato, now Dr. Sato. When he was in high school, Sato attended a meditation ceremony. As he sat cross-legged for hours, his legs went numb. He realized that his blood circulation was being blocked, and being an avid fitness buff and weight lifter, he noticed that the sensation was similar to the "pump" he felt when he lifted weights.

Over the next several years, Sato experimented on himself. He tied bicycle tubes around various body parts, taking note of the effects. When he later broke his ankle in a ski accident, he exercised the leg

---

306 Masumeh Darvishi et al., "Effect of Aerobic Training with Blood Flow Restricting on Static Balance, Lower Extremity Strength, and Thigh Hypertrophy in Females with Multiple Sclerosis," *Report of Health Care Journal* 3, no. 2 (April 2017): 33–41, https://jrhc.marvdasht.iau.ir/article_2927.html.

307 Víctor M. Arce, Pablo Devesa, and Jesús Devesa, "Role of Growth Hormone (GH) in the Treatment on Neural Diseases: From Neuroprotection to Neural Repair," *Neuroscience Research* 76, no. 4 (August 2013): 179–86, https://doi.org/10.1016/j.neures.2013.03.014.

308 Raymond L. Hintz, "Growth Hormone: Uses and Abuses," *BMJ* 328 (April 15, 2004): 907, https://doi.org/10.1136/bmj.328.7445.907.

with his compression bands on. The speed of his recovery amazed his doctors. To their surprise, they found that there was no atrophy in his leg when his cast came off.

After years of study and experimentation, Sato discovered that carefully restricting his blood flow improved his ability to train and recover.

By the way, I am *not* recommending that you tie bike tubes around parts of your body or experiment on yourself in any other strange ways. It makes for an amazing story, but fortunately, there are now more systematic, less potentially damaging ways to get the benefits of this practice.

It turns out that BFR works by stimulating the release of HGH. For weight lifters like Sato, that means more muscle mass and faster recovery times. For *everyone*, it means making your brain more resilient to stress, damage, and injury. Increased growth hormone means faster metabolism and more energy;[309] greater production of various immune cells and proteins necessary for healthy immune function;[310] improved cognitive functions such as memory, attention, and learning;[311] *and* an increased ability to prevent or slow down the progression of conditions that affect the brain, such as neurodegenerative diseases like amyotrophic lateral sclerosis (ALS) or Parkinson's disease, as well as injuries like stroke or head injury.[312]

---

309 Joshua E. Brinkman et al., *Physiology, Growth Hormone* (Treasure Island, FL: StatPearls Publishing, 2023), https://www.ncbi.nlm.nih.gov/books/NBK482141/.

310 Mohamed Hamdy Elkarow and Amr Hamdy, "A Suggested Role of Human Growth Hormone in Control of the COVID-19 Pandemic," *Frontiers in Endocrinology* 11 (November 8, 2020), https://doi.org/10.3389/fendo.2020.569633.

311 Daniel G. Blackmore and Michael J. Waters, "The Multiple Roles of GH in Neural Ageing and Injury," *Frontiers in Neuroscience* 17 (March 2023), https://doi.org/10.3389/fnins.2023.1082449; Fred Nyberg and Mathias Hallberg, "Growth Hormone and Cognitive Function," *Nature Reviews Endocrinology* 9 (April 30, 2013): 357–65, https://doi.org/10.1038/nrendo.2013.78; and Lin Kooi Ong et al., "Growth Hormone Improves Cognitive Function after Experimental Stroke," *Stroke* 49, no. 5 (2018): 1257–66, https://doi.org/10.1161/STROKEAHA.117.020557.

312 Jin-Young Chung et al., "The Neuroprotective Effects of Human Growth Hormone as a Potential Treatment for Amyotrophic Lateral Sclerosis," *Neural Regeneration Research* 10, no. 8 (August 2015): 1201–203, https://doi.org/10.4103%2F1673-5374.162690; Imma Castilla-Cortázar et al., "Is Insulin-Like Growth Factor-1 Involved in Parkinson's Disease Development?," *Journal of Translational Medicine* 18 (February 11, 2020), 70, https://doi.org/10.1186/s12967-020-02223-0; Shuyuan Huang et al., "Research Progress on the Role of Hormones in Ischemic Stroke," *Frontiers in Immunology* 13 (December 6, 2022), https://doi.org/10.3389/fimmu.2022.1062977; and P. Reimunde et al., "Effects of Growth Hormone (GH) Replacement and Cognitive Rehabilitation in Patients with Cognitive Disorders after Traumatic Brain Injury," *Brain Injury* 25, no. 1 (2011): 65–73, https://doi.org/10.3109/02699052.2010.536196.

And BFR can also bioaccelerate the benefits of exercising for non-athletes and people with inflammation-related conditions.

Exercise with BFR: All the Benefits

Remember in Chapter Four, when we talked about the many mental health benefits of exercise—especially interval training? One of the potential barriers we talked about in that chapter was the difficulty of jumping straight into high-intensity physical activity. BFR can help overcome that barrier. Recent research suggests that **low-intensity exercise *with* BFR has the same mood-boosting effects as high-intensity exercise without it.**[313]

Admittedly, that study involved young, highly trained athletes. But the benefits of exercise with BFR go way, way beyond athletes. For example, strength training has long been used for stroke survivors to improve strength and rebuild lost functionality. Now, studies have found that **strength training with BFR after a stroke significantly increases neuroprotective factors in the blood, compared to strength training alone.**[314] That means faster and more complete recovery and better protection against future strokes.

The benefits of exercising with BFR almost seem too good to be true in some cases. One study, for example, found that **older women who walked on a treadmill *with* BFR while doing mental exercises had a higher quality of life, better sleep, lower body-fat percentages, better knee extension, higher rates of neuroprotective factors, and higher overall mood**—even compared to other women who walked the same amount and did the same mental exercises.[315]

---

313 Julio Cesar Gomes da Silva et al., "Aerobic Exercise with Blood Flow Restriction Affects Mood State in a Similar Fashion to High Intensity Interval Exercise," *Physiology & Behavior* 211 (November 2019): 112677, https://doi.org/10.1016/j.physbeh.2019.112677.

314 Xiaochen Du et al., "The Effects of Low-Intensity Resistance Training with or without Blood Flow Restriction on Serum BDNF, VEGF and Perception in Patients with Post-Stroke Depression," *Neuroendocrinology Letters* 42, no. 4 (2021): 229–35, https://pubmed.ncbi.nlm.nih.gov/34436843/.

315 Amir Kargaran et al., "Effects of Dual-Task Training with Blood Flow Restriction on Cognitive Functions, Muscle Quality, and Circulatory Biomarkers in Elderly Women," *Physiology & Behavior* 239 (October 1, 2021): 113500, https://doi.org/10.1016/j.physbeh.2021.113500.

Okay, I know. You get it. But just one more because it's so exciting. Remember how I told you about the connection between hypertension and mental health symptoms in Chapter Four? How exercise helps reduce inflammation? Well, a 2018 study found that for older women with hypertension, low-impact exercise with BFR increased their antioxidant levels and reduced oxidative stress. Less inflammation, less damage.[316]

Just to cap it all off, BFR may even reduce jet lag![317]

Compared to medications, therapy, or even cold plunging, walking on a treadmill with a blood pressure cuff on is amazingly accessible. Just don't try it alone. At least at first, you need an expert to help you know just how much restriction to use, how to apply it, and how intensely you should be exercising.

And now...onto our last bioaccelerator, and one of the most technologically exciting: biofeedback.

Retrain Your Stress Response

One of the reasons it's so difficult to change your responses to long-term stress is that they happen unconsciously, outside of your conscious awareness. Often, you don't even know that your stress response has kicked on.

Biofeedback and *neurofeedback* are technologies that make your unconscious responses visible so that you can actively change them.

It's like learning a new skill. Imagine you're trying to learn wood carving. You start out with a block of wood and start cutting away pieces. How do you know you're doing it right? You keep looking at the block of wood and seeing if it looks the way you want. You

316 Angélica Barili et al., "Acute Responses of Hemodynamic and Oxidative Stress Parameters to Aerobic Exercise with Blood Flow Restriction in Hypertensive Elderly Women," *Molecular Biology Reports* 45 (2018): 1099–109, https://doi.org/10.1007/s11033-018-4261-1.

317 Maria Kotopoulea Nikolaidi et al., "The Potential of Blood Flow Restriction Exercise to Overcome Jetlag: Important Implications for Tokyo 2020," *Medicina Dello Sport* 74, no. 3 (September 2021): 435–40, https://doi.org/10.23736/S0025-7826.21.03993-4.

make a few cuts and evaluate, then make a few more cuts and evaluate again.

And if you have an expert to look at the block of wood with you and make suggestions about how to improve your cuts, all the better.

That's what biofeedback and neurofeedback do: they turn your stress response from something mysterious and hard to control into visible feedback you can understand and manage. And working with an expert helps you interpret the feedback and make the most impactful behavior changes to shift your experience.

Biofeedback

Biofeedback is a general term for a practice that trains you to control your own physiological processes.

Physiological processes is just science-speak for stuff that happens inside your body, whether that's digestion, respiration, or the immune response. Biofeedback makes specific physiological processes more conscious so that you can learn to control them.

Specifically, biofeedback lets you control your body's unconscious, or autonomic, responses, such as heart rate or sweating. The person undergoing biofeedback is hooked up to a monitor and trained to use specific techniques to change the outcomes on the monitor. For example, they might be trained to slow their breathing to bring down their heart rate. Or they might learn new stress management techniques that reduce their sweating (anxiety) response.

And voilà! They've learned to control a physiological process that was previously totally unconscious.

Biofeedback that focuses on slowing or controlling heart rate is especially common and important because heart rate is such a strong indicator of stress and anxiety. When you're in fight-or-flight, your heart rate spikes up. When you live with stress over long periods, your heart rate can stay elevated even when the "danger" is long gone.

And it's not just the rate that matters. New science has discovered a connection between stress and heart rate *variability*. If your heart rate is how fast or slow your heart is beating, heart rate variability (HRV) is when your heart rate varies slightly between each beat. Sometimes the space between beats is longer, sometimes shorter. Your heart rate isn't constant. High variability means high adaptability, which is good, whereas low variability means rigidity and is a sign of distress.

What's fascinating is that even though HRV is so miniscule that it can only be measured by high-tech devices, low HRV has been linked to a lot of negative health outcomes, from heart conditions to depression and anxiety.[318] It's also been linked to the decrease in working memory common in people with depression, and it appears to be strongly correlated with long-term stress.[319]

HRV biofeedback, then, is biofeedback that shows you the variability in your heart rate, not just the speed, and teaches you to control or reduce it through behaviors like breathing patterns and thoughts.

THE PROMISE OF HRV BIOFEEDBACK

Heart rate variability biofeedback is especially promising for people living with chronic, inflammation-related conditions.

Migraine sufferers trained with HRV biofeedback used fewer painkillers and experienced less migraine-related depression after treatment.[320] People with concussions who got just eleven sessions of HRV bio-

---

318 Cleveland Clinic, "Heart Rate Variability (HRV)," Health Library, September 1, 2021, https://my.clevelandclinic.org/health/symptoms/21773-heart-rate-variability-hrv.

319 Deokjong Lee et al., "Associations between Heart Rate Variability and Brain Activity during a Working Memory Task: A Primary Electroencephalogram Study on Depression and Anxiety Disorder," *Brain Sciences* 12, no. 2 (January 28, 2022): 172, https://doi.org/10.3390/brainsci12020172; and Hye-Geum Kim et al., "Stress and Heart-Rate Variability: A Meta-Analysis and Review of the Literature," *Psychiatry Investigation* 15, no. 3 (2018): 235–45, https://doi.org/10.30773/pi.2017.08.17.

320 Ami Cuneo et al., "The Utility of a Novel, Combined Biofeedback-Virtual Reality Device as Add-On Treatment for Chronic Migraine: A Randomized Pilot Study," *Clinical Journal of Pain* 39, no. 6 (June 2023): 286–96, https://doi.org/10.1097/ajp.0000000000001114.

feedback showed improvements in their HRV and in their cognitive symptoms and emotional functioning, along with reductions in headaches, dizziness, and sleep problems.[321]

HRV biofeedback has been shown to reduce depression and insomnia symptoms in people with major depressive disorder (MDD) and, interestingly, also reduced depression scores in people who received biofeedback treatment for heart disease.[322]

Perhaps most amazingly, at least one study suggests that HRV biofeedback can achieve a *complete elimination* of PTSD symptoms, including nightmares, dissociation, avoidance behaviors, and negative mood. In that study, which combined biofeedback with cognitive behavioral therapy in 30 adults with PTSD, *not one* of the participants still met the definition of even *having* PTSD after the treatment. That's how much their symptoms had improved.[323]

Neurofeedback (EEG Biofeedback)

Neurofeedback is biofeedback for your brain waves. It's also called EEG biofeedback because it uses an electroencephalogram (EEG), a machine that measures the electrical pulses in your brain.

Your brain is like a symphony of activity. If you've ever seen pictures of brain scans, you've seen the symphony in action. You'll

---

321 Leah D. Talbert et al., "A Systematic Review of Heart Rate Variability (HRV) Biofeedback Treatment following Traumatic Brain Injury (TBI)," *Brain Injury* 37, no. 7 (2023): 635–42, https://doi.org/10.1080/o 2699052.2023.2208880.

322 I-Mei Lin et al., "Heart Rate Variability Biofeedback Increased Autonomic Activation and Improved Symptoms of Depression and Insomnia among Patients with Major Depression Disorder," *Clinical Psychopharmacology and Neuroscience* 17, no. 2 (2019): 222–32, https://doi.org/10.9758/ cpn.2019.17.2.222; and Li-Ching Yu et al., "One-Year Cardiovascular Prognosis of the Randomized, Controlled, Short-Term Heart Rate Variability Biofeedback among Patients with Coronary Artery Disease," *International Journal of Behavioral Medicine* 25 (January 2018): 271–82, https://doi.org/10.1007/ s12529-017-9707-7.

323 Shawn R. Criswell, Richard Sherman, and Stanley Krippner, "Cognitive Behavioral Therapy with Heart Rate Variability Biofeedback for Adults with Persistent Noncombat-Related Posttraumatic Stress Disorder," *Permanente Journal* 22, no. 4 (December 1, 2018), https://doi.org/10.7812/TPP/17-207.

see a region at the back of the brain light up, then fade as another area bursts into activity, and then another. These bursts of activity are brain waves: the electrical pulses inside our brains that make up our thoughts, feelings, and experiences.

And just like a symphony, different types of brain waves create different effects in our brains and bodies. Some are like cellos, soothing and slow, firing when we're sleepy or calm. Others are like trumpets, blaring awake in moments of anxiety or stress.

Each type of brain wave is related to different mental and emotional states. If you're anxious, for example, you probably have increased beta waves. If you're sleepy, you're more likely in an alpha and theta brain wave state. Most of the time, we think of our brain waves as something we can't control. After all, they are microsecond electrical impulses happening inside our skulls.

Neurofeedback allows you to become the conductor of your own brain wave symphony. It trains you to be able to calm the blaring trumpets and awaken the soothing cellos. By watching the response of your own brain waves in real time via the EEG, you learn methods for calming and soothing yourself, actually changing the patterns of your own brain.

Like biofeedback, neurofeedback has been shown to treat a surprising range of disorders including depression, anorexia, dyslexia, ADD, ADHD, schizophrenia, substance use disorders, PTSD, and Alzheimer's disease.[324] One 2014 study found that EEG biofeedback improved functioning and lessened symptoms in people with autism spectrum disorder, while another in 2015 demonstrated improved cognitive functioning from EEG biofeedback in people with various types of dementia, including Alzheimer's.[325]

---

324 Lisa S. Panisch and Audrey Hang Hai, "The Effectiveness of Using Neurofeedback in the Treatment of Post-Traumatic Stress Disorder: A Systematic Review," *Trauma, Violence, and Abuse* 21, no. 3 (2020): 541–50, https://doi.org/10.1177/1524838018781103; and Javier Vigil Morant, "Neurotherapies and Alzheimer: A Protocol Oriented Review," *NeuroRegulation* 4, no. 2 (2017): 79–94, https://doi.org/10.15540/nr.4.2.79.

325 Robert Coben et al., "Connectivity-Guided EEG Biofeedback for Autism Spectrum Disorder: Evidence of Neurophysiological Changes," *NeuroRegulation* 1, no. 2 (2014): 109–130, https://doi.org/10.15540/nr.1.2.109; and Nancy L. Wigton and Genomary Krigbaum, "A Review of qEEG-Guided Neurofeedback," *NeuroRegulation* 2, no. 3 (2015): 149–55, https://doi.org/10.15540/nr.2.3.149.

Even athletes are getting into the feedback game, so to speak. The Italian national soccer team used a combination of biofeedback and neurofeedback to optimize their performance before their 2006 World Cup victory. The practices helped them maintain optimal breathing patterns, relax their muscles, control their heart rates, and keep their brains in the relaxed alpha zone. In other words, they reduced their natural, unconscious responses to the overwhelming stress of being on the world stage.[326]

The body's stress responses are similar, whether you're running out onto the field in front of tens of thousands of screaming fans or living with chronic stress from early trauma or inflammatory disease. Biofeedback and neurofeedback make those responses visible so you can train and overcome them.

NEW TECH TO RETRAIN THE BRAIN

Researchers continue to develop new technologies that directly retrain your brain to reduce inflammation and the symptoms of stress and trauma. In many cases, these technologies are passive: you can just sit and let them work. Some of these may be less accessible than the accelerators I introduced earlier, but if you can access them, they are definitely worth looking into.

Pulsating Electromagnetic Fields (PEMF)

Scientists studying how to help people recover from stroke have started to see exciting neuroprotective results from PEMF. PEMF can reduce the area of the brain that's affected and decrease the pro-

---

326 Vietta Wilson, Erik Peper, and Donald Moss, "'The Mind Room' in Italian Soccer Training: The Use of Biofeedback and Neurofeedback for Optimum Performance," *Biofeedback* 34, no. 3 (Fall 2006): 79–81, https://www.researchgate.net/publication/259558691_The_Mind_Room_in_Italian_soccer_training_The_use_of_biofeedback_and_neurofeedback_for_optimum_performance.

inflammatory response that often follows a stroke.[327] One patient suffering from long COVID-19 was given a PEMF intervention and saw their symptoms resolve *the next day*.[328] At six months, the symptoms had still not returned. That is an accelerator, for sure!

PEMF, or pulsating electromagnetic fields, works by sending magnetic energy into the brain. The magnetic energy changes the patterns of brain waves without any intervention from you. Some PEMF can be done using a mat you sit or lie down on or with a PEMF headband. There are even PEMF products you can use at home. Other types of PEMF require more substantial equipment and take place in a clinical setting.

Transcranial Magnetic Stimulation (TMS)

Although these are some of the more strange-sounding technologies in this chapter, both PEMF and TMS have been shown to decrease inflammation, and both have been studied as treatments for depression.[329] TMS in particular has been shown to improve cognition and reduce neurological symptoms across multiple kinds of dementia, and multiple studies suggest it is effective in treating substance use disorders as well.[330]

The word *transcranial* means "across the skull." So while TMS

---

327 Fioravante Capone et al., "Pulsed Electromagnetic Fields: A Novel Attractive Therapeutic Opportunity for Neuroprotection after Acute Cerebral Ischemia," *Neuromodulation* 25, no. 8 (December 2022): 1240–47, https://doi.org/10.1111/ner.13489.

328 Laura V. Schaefer and Frank N. Bittmann, "Case Report: Individualized Pulsed Electromagnetic Field Therapy in a Long COVID Patient Using the Adaptive Force as Biomarker," *Frontiers in Medicine* 9 (January 11, 2023), https://doi.org/10.3389/fmed.2022.879971.

329 Hiroshi Tateishi, Yoshito Mizoguchi, and Akira Monji, "Is the Therapeutic Mechanism of Repetitive Transcranial Magnetic Stimulation in Cognitive Dysfunctions of Depression Related to the Neuroinflammatory Processes in Depression?," *Frontiers in Psychiatry* 13 (February 23, 2022), https://doi.org/10.3389/fpsyt.2022.834425.

330 Greg J. Elder and John-Paul Taylor, "Transcranial Magnetic Stimulation and Transcranial Direct Current Stimulation: Treatments for Cognitive and Neuropsychiatric Symptoms in the Neurodegenerative Dementias?," *Alzheimer's Research & Therapy* 6 (November 10, 2014): 74, https://doi.org/10.1186/s13195-014-0074-1; and David A. Gorelick, Abraham Zangen, and Mark S. George, "Transcranial Magnetic Stimulation in the Treatment of Substance Addiction," *Annals of the New York Academy of Sciences* 1327, no. 1 (October 2014): 79–93, https://doi.org/10.1111/nyas.12479.

also sends magnetic fields into the brain, the process is a little different from PEMF. Instead of wearable technologies or mats, TMS uses an MRI machine to allow the magnetic field to pass all the way through the brain. Because of this, you can only access TMS through a clinic.

TMS has been shown to be a powerful tool against depression. Most incredibly of all, TMS has been found to increase brain activity in *coma* patients. Very few effective treatments exist for people in a so-called persistent vegetative state (a long-term coma), but TMS shows promise. It appears to increase conscious brain function in these patients, and it may help people recover from all kinds of "disturbances of consciousness," or periods of coma.[331]

TMS has even been effective in helping to reduce symptoms of psychiatric disorders like bipolar disorder and schizophrenia.[332] Given that these are not only inflammation-related conditions but are considered extremely hard to treat and offer very few effective therapies, the positive results from these new studies are hopeful indeed.

Vagus Nerve Stimulation

There are devices that can stimulate your vagus nerve directly through the skin. Called *transcutaneous devices* (*trans* meaning "across" and *cutaneous* referring to the skin), some look like fancy earbuds, while others use contacts on the thin skin of your wrist. Despite their unassuming appearance, these devices deliver surprising anti-inflammatory effects, including reducing those pro-inflammatory cytokines we talked about earlier.[333] More recently, this treatment has

---

331 Xiao-Hua Zhang et al., "The Clinical Effect of Repetitive Transcranial Magnetic Stimulation on the Disturbance of Consciousness in Patients in a Vegetative State," *Frontiers in Neuroscience* 15 (April 29, 2021), https://doi.org/10.3389/fnins.2021.647517.

332 F. S. Bersani et al., "Deep Transcranial Magnetic Stimulation as a Treatment for Psychiatric Disorders: A Comprehensive Review," *European Psychiatry* 28, no. 1 (2013): 30–39, https://doi.org/10.1016/j.eurpsy.2012.02.006.

333 Yu Xue Zhao et al., "Transcutaneous Auricular Vagus Nerve Stimulation Protects Endotoxemic Rat from Lipopolysaccharide-Induced Inflammation," *Evidence-Based Complementary and Alternative Medicine* 2012 (December 29, 2012): 627023, https://doi.org/10.1155/2012/627023.

been proposed as a new method for treating inflammatory diseases from polycystic ovary syndrome to COVID-19.[334]

We've talked about the parasympathetic nervous system a lot (it's the "rest-and-digest" system, the opposite of fight-or-flight). This part of your nervous system is regulated by your vagus nerve, which runs all the way from your brain to your gut. The vagus nerve is why you get that "gut feeling" when something seems off.

Practices like meditation and psychotherapy "tone" your vagus nerve so that you can stay in and bounce back to your parasympathetic system faster and more easily. Now it turns out you can use technology to bioaccelerate that effect.

Although direct vagus nerve stimulation is new enough that it's still seen as "alternative" medicine by some, the evidence for its benefits suggests it is another potential ally against chronic inflammation.

Tempo and Rhythm

In Chapter Eight, we talked about the nervous-system resetting effects of social interaction. Well, one of the benefits of being social creatures is that other people's moods can change our own. Just being around calm people makes us feel calmer—and lowers inflammation. We respond naturally to people and rhythms in our surroundings. The tempo of music in a café can cause our heart rate and breathing to speed up or slow down.[335] Even in the womb, a pregnant mother's heartbeat facilitates neural development in a growing baby.[336]

The *doppel* wearable device lightly pulses a slow tempo (like the

---

334 Shike Zhang et al., "Transcutaneous Auricular Vagus Nerve Stimulation as a Potential Novel Treatment for Polycystic Ovary Syndrome," *Scientific Reports* 13 (May 12, 2023): 7721, https://doi.org/10.1038/s41598-023-34746-z; and Fernando Mendes Sant'Anna et al., "Auricular Vagus Nerve Stimulation: A New Option to Treat Inflammation in COVID-19?," *Revista da Associacao Medica Brasileira* 69, no. 6 (2023), https://doi.org/10.1590/1806-9282.20230345.

335 Sylvia D. Kreibig, "Autonomic Nervous System Activity in Emotion: A Review," *Biological Psychology* 84, no. 3 (July 2010): 394–421, https://doi.org/10.1016/j.biopsycho.2010.03.010.

336 Ruth Feldman, "Parent–Infant Synchrony: Biological Foundations and Developmental Outcomes," *Current Directions in Psychological Science* 16, no. 6 (2007): 340–45, https://doi.org/10.1111/j.1467-8721.2007.00532.x.

heartbeat of a nearby friend) on your wrist throughout the day. The device can be calming even in circumstances that would make anyone nervous. Like the study that looked at people who were preparing to give a speech. Half wore a doppel device on their wrist that was set at a pace about 20 percent lower than their own heart rate. The doppel group felt a lot less anxiety, and their physical measures of stress were lower.[337]

The real kicker about this study is that the doppel group only had the device turned on for about *five minutes* prior to giving their speech. I'd try almost anything that made me feel better about public speaking that quickly!

Bilateral Stimulation

Just for fun, let's end with the simplest, most accessible "technology" of all: your own body.

Remember how we talked about EMDR in Chapter Nine? Moving the eyes back and forth (like what naturally happens during REM sleep) tells the parasympathetic nervous system to kick in and the fight-or-flight response to calm down. Well, scientists are finding out that something called *bilateral stimulation* (which just means touching or moving both sides of the body) can accomplish the same thing.

Back-and-forth stimulation between the right and left sides of the brain has a calming effect on the nervous system. What's amazing is that "stimulation" doesn't have to mean anything fancy. It can be as simple as moving your arm. The left arm activates the right brain. The right arm activates the left brain.

Put one hand on each knee. First, tap the left knee with your left hand. Then tap the right knee with your right hand. Repeat: left, right, left, and so on. It's that crazy simple.

As far as tech goes, a device that provides a consistent tempo back

---

337 Ruben T. Azevedo et al., "The Calming Effect of a New Wearable Device during the Anticipation of Public Speech," *Scientific Reports* 7 (May 23, 2017): 2285, https://doi.org/10.1038/s41598-017-02274-2.

and forth can work wonders. Like the TouchPoint device that pulses on the inside of each wrist—first one wrist, then the other. Research shows that when people use the TouchPoint while under stress, their stress levels went down a lot more than the control group, and a saliva test showed that they didn't just "feel better." Their levels of the stress hormone cortisol were also lower.[338]

A little buzz on this wrist, and then a little buzz on the other, and the body's natural anti-stress systems came to the rescue. Now *that's* what I call a bioaccelerator.

RECOMMENDATIONS

You've heard it so many times now, you can probably say it with me: "If it's powerful enough to help, it's powerful enough to hurt." These bioaccelerators, as promising as they are, are no exception to that rule.

Here's how to make good choices.

LOOK AT EVIDENCE AND REPUTATION

The good news is that personal wellness and optimal health are becoming increasingly important to people around the world. The not-as-good news is that there are plenty of people looking to cash in on that movement.

As you look around for ways to access these bioaccelerators, you might see options that seem too good to be true. They probably are.

Your mental health is worth taking the time to do your research. Look for evidence-based practices (like the ones I've introduced you to in this chapter). Learn everything you can about the technologies you're interested in. Are they supported by clinical data? Has anyone

---

338 Ernesto Cesar Pinto Leal-Junior et al., "A Triple-Blind, Placebo-Controlled Randomized Trial of the Effect of Bilateral Alternating Somatosensory Stimulation on Reducing Stress-Related Cortisol and Anxiety during and after the Trier Social Stress Test," *Journal of Biotechnology and Biomedical Science* 2, no. 1 (June 25, 2019): 22–30, https://doi.org/10.14302/issn.2576-6694.jbbs-19-2784.

published studies? You can ask your doctor or a friend with a science background to help you make sense of the research.

How you access a given technology also matters. Remember when I talked about psychedelics, I said that you need to look for a medical clinic, not a day spa? The same is true here. Find out the reputation of the provider you want to try. Does the clinic have reviews? If you're using a technology you can bring home, like a PEMF mat, is the manufacturer reputable? What are others saying about them? What appears to be the "same" technology can be very different depending on who manufactures it or how it's being delivered.

It's always a good idea to do some research before spending money on a product. When the product can profoundly influence your brain and body, it's worth taking the time to investigate it thoroughly.

But Is It for Real?

All information is not created equal, and it can be hard to know which claims about health and wellness technologies are really supported by the evidence.

Here are a few tips to keep in mind while you're doing your research:

1. Check out the source of the information. Is it coming from a scientific journal? Is the source a reporter for a well-respected newspaper? Have they written on this topic or related topics before?
2. Look at how (and whether) they give credit for ideas. Does the article you're reading cite sources? Does it point you to other places to find more information?
3. Take time into account. When was the information published? Is it recent? Does it reflect current ideas about the topic?
4. Think about bias. Does the author only provide one point of view or try to push you toward believing something in particular? Do they report on potential downsides or only the benefits or positive information (or vice versa)?

COMBINE THERAPIES FOR GREATER BENEFIT

Each of these bioaccelerating technologies alone can be a potent force for change. But combining things can magnify the changes and improvements beyond what each alone can deliver.

At Mindeo® brain fitness centers, for example, I have brought together the best evidence-supported technologies and methods and made it simple to get the magnified benefits that come from combining them into a streamlined experience. Our team leads individuals through guided SynapFit™ sessions that are convenient and accessible.

Likewise, you could combine neurofeedback sessions, light therapy and cold therapy at home to get a bigger-than-one-alone impact.

My vision is a future in which every person is empowered to achieve optimal brain fitness and to see and experience the world through a more positive lens, with a balanced mood, ample energy, and great cognitive ability. That's what I call optimal brain fitness.

New science continues to make it more and more possible for everyone to enjoy a better level of brain fitness and a better life, and because these new insights can get stuck in the lab, I'll continue to work to bring the best tools and information to everyone!

PUTTING IT ALL TOGETHER

Let's visit Ash one more time.

Ash's story is striking. When I first met them, Ash had been suffering symptoms of depression for decades. They had been on and off of SSRIs. Their migraines were worse than ever, and they lived with an almost unmanageable burden of chronic stress. Ash wasn't eating or sleeping well and was finding it harder and harder to push through each day.

I bet, if you are reading this book, some of Ash's symptoms and struggles sound familiar. Maybe some of Camilla's, Stephanie's, or Jadyn's do too.

Ash is also remarkable because of the dedication they put into getting well. Ash used tools from every part of this book, from sleep hygiene to supplements to high-tech interventions.

When Ash's sleep problems got so bad they were barely able to work, they came to Mindeo. There, they did regular SynapFit sessions consisting of interval movement combined with bioaccelerating technologies.

After eight weeks, Ash had more energy than they could remember having since they were a teenager. They were sleeping through the night. Their mood felt balanced, and they hadn't had a migraine since the second week of their brain fitness program.

They felt the energy and space in their life to make plans with friends and to try therapy again, and this time it felt like an exciting step into exploring what's important to them. Plus, they felt less worn down by work travel and felt ready for the next challenge that appears.

And that, in the end, is why I do this work. When someone like Ash discovers tools, uses them, and thrives—that's what it's all about.

Best of all, Ash is not alone. These technologies and therapies—they work. When you use approaches that directly reduce inflammation and mend your brain by speeding up your body's own natural healing processes, you can get better.

For me, that's not just lip service. It's the story of my own life. It's how I gave myself the gift of a better life—and how you can do the same.

TL;DR

→ New technologies have been developed that can create significant changes quickly and use your body's own healing abilities to help you feel better faster.

→ When you're dealing with mental health issues, the damage from inflammation can overpower your body's ability to repair itself. Bioaccelerators can help tip the balance, increasing your *rate of repair*.

→ Some bioaccelerating technologies amp up environmental elements (like light or oxygen) to give your body a concentrated dose of what it needs, while others (like PEMF and biofeedback) retrain your systems to get them back in balance.

→ Researchers are constantly studying new technologies to improve brain function, reduce mental health symptoms, and fight inflammation. Some of these new technologies may have the ability to repair the brain quickly and noninvasively.

→ Now is an amazing time to be starting your brain-health journey. New technologies and new research are coming out every year. More options and more tools are available than ever before.

CONCLUSION

Wow. We have covered a lot of ground here. Congratulations for getting here and for making the commitment to improve your own mental health and well-being.

Before we part company, there are a few key takeaway points I want to leave you with.

If you remember nothing else from this book, remember this: "better" is out there.

For me, what's been most amazing about this journey is that I don't just feel "better" than I did after my accident. I feel better *than I ever have.* Even though I have a chronic version of post-concussion syndrome that I'll be managing for the rest of my life, my quality of life is *still* better than it was before I got injured. That's thanks to the methods I've outlined in this book.

That's the biggie. The most important thing to take away. *You can feel better.*

The other is that new ways to feel better are being discovered all the time.

Almost every day, exciting new science is showing us how inflammation is related to mental health—and new ways to prevent, manage, treat, and even reverse inflammation-related damage. That's something to celebrate, for anyone with a brain. (Which means all of us!)

While we're at it, here are a few more critical points to carry with you:

- Inflammation is an important part of your body's response to injury and illness, but when it becomes chronic or flares out of control, it can cause problems ranging from anxiety and brain fog, to fatigue and sleeplessness, to Alzheimer's disease and dementia.

- All kinds of stress—including chronic stressors like overwhelming work schedules and acute stressors like traumatic events—can turn on the inflammation cycle and, over time, contribute to inflammation-related conditions and symptoms.

- Any symptoms you're experiencing now could be related to stressors or life events years or even decades in the past, some of which you may not even remember.

- Lifestyle changes can have powerful, long-term effects on inflammation and mental health, and making small changes can have big impacts.

- Therapy and medication can be great tools in your mental health toolbox, but they're not all created equal, and some can have substantial side effects.

- Always ask *why* you're using or being given a particular medication, supplement, or other treatment, *what* it will do for you, and *how long* you can expect to need it.

- Don't just accept the "same old, same old" when it comes to your own quality of life. There is so much more out there that can help you, with new methods being pioneered every day. Using this book as your guide, take your mental health into your own hands.

Now that you've got all the *information* you need, what's next? That's simple. Do just one thing.

Choose *one* lifestyle change you want to try out, like eating more blueberries and fewer cookies. Reclaim your bedtime routine or cut out afternoon coffee so you can sleep better. Or check out a bioaccelerator, like setting up an appointment to try out exercise with oxygen therapy or getting yourself a red light for those dark days of winter.

Select one of the many options I've laid out for you here and just...give it a try.

You don't have to do everything at once. You don't have to change your whole life overnight. If you have inflammation-related mental health challenges, they probably didn't develop all at once. Most likely, it took years for the inflammation to build up to where it is now.

So give yourself a break. Give yourself time to improve. Commit to yourself by choosing something you feel confident you can do and starting there.

And you know what? Once you've done one thing, *take time to celebrate it*. You did something to improve your own mental health and well-being. That's worth recognizing.

I have been where you are. I have spent months on the couch, too fatigued and brain-fogged to live my life. I have felt the devastation of inflammatory disease and the chronic mental health problems that can come with it.

Which is why I can say with certainty: it's worth the work to get to the other side.

As I'm writing this last message to you, I'm also in the middle of expanding and growing Mindeo, my brain fitness business. I am constantly juggling important priorities, from supporting the team to meeting with partners, to catching up on the latest research in brain science.

Every day, I remember how not so long ago I would have been unable to do any of these things. That's what I think about when I see clients come into the center who are fatigued, anxious, or otherwise not able to live the lives they want—people who are where I was.

When those clients come in, I can't help smiling. Because now I know what's possible and how their quality of life can change. And now, with the information in this book, you have what you need to get started on that path as well.

Which is another way of saying: go get some rest, take a walk, plant your garden, or make that appointment to try out sensory deprivation or biofeedback. Take your first step toward reclaiming your own well-being.

Better is out there.

ACKNOWLEDGMENTS

This book would not have been possible without the incredible support, expertise, and insight of a number of people. In particular, we have relied on these individuals to:

- Review the book for scientific and clinical accuracy
- Identify the key areas that we should cover and which issues impacted the most people
- Help us understand the human impact of mental health issues
- Ensure that the individuals and groups discussed in the book are represented accurately and with sensitivity

We would especially like to thank:

- Dr. Christopher Hughes, MD, Medical Director of the Neuro ICU and Chief of Anesthesiology for Critical Care Medicine at Vanderbilt University Medical Center, as well as Medical Advisor to Mindeo brain fitness centers. Thank you for your complete and thorough review of the science and your commitment to accuracy and scientific rigor.
- Daniel Smith, PhD, Medical Physicist. Thank you for your scien-

tific review and for the candid feedback on the readability of the scientific information in the book.

- Dr. Cory Funk, PhD, Senior Research Scientist at the Hood-Price Lab, and Scientific Advisor to Mindeo. Thank you for helping us understand the fundamental neurobiology we needed for the book, especially the immunological functions in the brain.
- Somi Panday, MPH, BSN, Nurse and Nursing Researcher. Thank you for your very thorough literature review and your assistance in locating the many studies cited in the book.
- Vicki Lopez, MA, LMHC, Therapist. Thank you for help in accurately characterizing and representing mental health issues.
- Nicholas Starbuck, BPsychSC, family member. Thank you for your assistance in understanding the stress and health impacts that minorities, underrepresented groups, and socioeconomically disadvantaged groups experience.
- The clients whose stories informed the book's characters. Your struggles and experiences both inspired this book and made it more relatable for others with similar struggles.
- The vast group of research scientists, clinicians, and their colleagues who have contributed so much knowledge to the literature, across the hundreds of papers we read. We're beyond grateful for the work you do, and the openness with which your findings are shared. Without researchers doing this work tirelessly behind the scenes, the knowledge shared in this book would not exist.
- Mark Gardett, writer. Thank you for your commitment and follow-through on writing and editorial support, major contributions to the structure of the book and the characters therein, and substantial reworking and editing of the text. It wouldn't have been possible to create this book without your help.

Note: Perplexity.ai was used to supplement the manual scientific research process. It was used to point out relevant studies that were missed in the initial search and cross-referencing process. We are grateful for this tool's effectiveness.

www.ingramcontent.com/pod-product-compliance
Lightning Source LLC
Chambersburg PA
CBHW031140020426
42333CB00013B/462